LOW GLYCEMIC INDEX DIET 2025

110 Healthy and Tasty Recipes Reach Your Ideal Weight, the Secret to Sustained Wellbeing

KLARLOCK

DISCLAIMER

This book aims to provide useful and informative material on the topics covered in the publication. It is sold with the understanding that the author and publisher are not engaged in rendering any personal medical, health care, or other professional services in the book. The reader should consult his or her physician, health care provider, or other competent professional before adopting any suggestions in this book or drawing any conclusions. The author and publisher expressly disclaim responsibility for any liability, loss, or risk, personal or otherwise, arising, directly or indirectly, from the use and application of any contents of this book.

NOTE

All the recipes in this book are designed for four people. For this quantity, the ingredients indicated in the recipes must be considered. If you need to change the portion, it is recommended to proportionally adjust the doses of the ingredients. It is also recommended to carefully follow the preparation and cooking instructions to obtain the best result. In the context of this book, when we refer to "a cup" as a unit of measurement for ingredients, we mean using a standard kitchen cup with a capacity of approximately 2 milliliters. It is essential to use a measuring cup to get the right quantities of ingredients. If you don't have a measuring cup, you can use a graduated measuring cup, making sure to correctly correspond to the proportions indicated. Here are some examples 1 Cup of flour 100 gr. 1 cup of rice 200 gr. 1 Cup of Quinoa 200 gr.

STABLE OF CONTENT

INTRODUCTION TO THE LOW GLYCEMIC INDEX DIET

UNDERSTANDING THE GLYCEMIC INDEX (GI)

IMPORTANCE OF THE GLYCEMIC INDEX IN THE DIET

BASICS OF THE GLYCEMIC INDEX

WHAT IS THE GLYCEMIC INDEX

HOW FOODS AFFECT BLOOD SUGAR LEVELS

HEALTH IMPACTS

IMPACT ON WEIGHT MANAGEMENT

GLYCEMIC INDEX AND METABOLIC HEALTH

IMPLEMENTATION OF THE GLYCEMIC INDEX DIET

CHOOSE FOODS WITH A LOW GLYCEMIC INDEX

CREATE BALANCED MEALS

MEAL PLANNING STRATEGIES

PRACTICAL TIPS FOR SUCCESS

BUY FOODS WITH A LOW GLYCEMIC INDEX

TIPS FOR COOKING AND PREPARING FOOD

EATING OUT WHILE FOLLOWING A LOW GLYCEMIC DIET

MANAGING CHALLENGES OVERCOMING COMMON OBSTACLES

ADAPT YOUR DIET TO DIFFERENT LIFESTYLES

ADDITIONAL INFORMATION ON THE GLYCEMIC INDEX

WHAT IS THE GLYCEMIC INDEX DIET

THE BENEFITS OF THE DIET

RECIPES APPETIZERS

73 WHOLE WHOLE BRUSCHETTAS WITH TOMATOES AND FRESH BASIL

75 WHOLE BREAD CROUTTONS WITH BLACK OLIVE PATÉ

77 CAPRESE SALAD WITH LIGHT MOZZARELLA AND CHERRY TOMATOES

79 RAW HAM WITH MELON SLICES

80 CARPACCIO OF COURGETTE WITH SKINNY CHEESE EXTRA VIRGIN OLIVE OIL

82 SEAFOOD SALAD WITH SHRIMP AND AVOCADO

84 GRILLED AUBERGINE ROLLS WITH LIGHT RICOTTA

86 PUMPKIN SOUP WITH ROSEMARY WHOLE CROUTTONS

88 ZUCCHINI AND CHICKPEA FLOUR FRITTERS

90 SALMON TARTARE WITH AVOCADO AND LIME

92 QUINOA SALAD WITH MIXED VEGETABLES

94 LIGHT MOZZARELLA IN CARROZZA WITH HOMEMADE MARINARA SAUCE

96 WHOLE CROUTTONS WITH RICOTTA AND HONEY

98 LEAN COOKED HAM AND FRESH FIGS

99 MARINATED OLIVES WITH AROMATIC HERBS AND LEMON

101 GRILLED AUBERGINES WITH DRIED TOMATOES AND FRESH BASIL

103 SMOKED SALMON CANAPES WITH SKINNY CREAM CHEESE

105 CANNELLINI BEAN SALAD WITH NATURAL TUNA AND RED ONION

107 CHICKEN BITES MARINATED WITH LEMON AND FRESH THYME

109 GUACAMOLE WITH RAW VEGETABLE STICKS

111 POMEGRANATE, ARUGULA AND LIGHT PARMESAN FLAKES SALAD

113 WHOLE CROUTTONS WITH PORCINI MUSHROOMS AND FRESH PARSLEY

115 CHICKEN MEATBALLS WITH HOMEMADE SWEET AND SOUR SAUCE

117 CHICKPEA SALAD WITH CHERRY TOMATOES AND CUCUMBERS

119 TOMATOES STUFFED WITH TUNA AND CAPERS

121 WHOLE CROUTTONS WITH RICOTTA, LEAN RAW HAM AND ARUGULA

123 SALMON TARTARE WITH AVOCADO AND MANGO

125 BAKED POTATOES WITH FRESH ROSEMARY AND GARLIC

127 WHOLE CROUTTONS WITH CONFIT TOMATOES AND BASIL PESTO

129 ORANGE, BLACK OLIVE AND FENNEL SALAD

131 WHOLE WHOLE CORN FRIES WITH LIGHT SPICY SAUCE

133 SMOKED SALMON AND LIGHT SPREADABLE CHEESE ROLLS

135 WHOLE CROUTTONS WITH LIGHT CREAM CHEESE AND ROASTED PEPPERS

137 CARPACCIO OF MIXED VEGETABLES WITH EXTRA VIRGIN OLIVE OIL AND LEMON

139 SALAD OF TOMATOES, LIGHT MOZZARELLA AND BASIL

141 WHOLE CROUTTONS WITH TUNA MOUSSE AND CAPERS

143 DRIED TOMATOES STUFFED WITH LIGHT RICOTTA AND BASIL

145 BAKED AUBERGINE MEATBALLS WITH TOMATO SAUCE WITHOUT ADDED SUGAR

147 WHOLEWHEAT PIE WITH SPINACH AND LIGHT RICOTTA

149 BROWN RICE SALAD WITH NATURAL TUNA, OLIVES AND CORN

RECIPES FIRST DISHES

152 WHOLE WHOLE SPAGHETTI WITH DRIED TOMATO PESTO

154 WHOLE WHOLE RISOTTO WITH MIXED MUSHROOMS

157 LENTIL SOUP WITH SPINACH

159 WHOLEWHEAT PENNE WITH FRESH TOMATO SAUCE

161 SPELLED WITH VEGETABLE SAUCE

163 BARLEY WITH COURGETTES AND TOMATOES

165 WILD RICE WITH STEAMED BROCCOLI

167 BUCKWHEAT LINGUINE WITH ARUGULA PESTO

169 AUBERGINES AND SPINACH LASAGNA

171 KONJAC TAGLIATELLE WITH TOMATO AND BASIL SAUCE

173 QUINOA WITH GRILLED VEGETABLES

175 WHOLE WHOLE RAVIOLI WITH RICOTTA AND SPINACH FILLING

177 PUMPKIN SPAGHETTI WITH TOMATO SAUCE

179 SWEET POTATO GNOCCHI WITH BASIL PESTO

181 SPELLED RISOTTO WITH SAFFRON AND ASPARAGUS

183 COURGETTE SPAGHETTI OMELETTE WITH TOMATOES

185 BASMATI RICE WITH VEGETABLE CURRY

187 WHOLE WHOLE COUSCOUS WITH CHICKPEAS AND TOMATO

189 OAT FETTUCCINE WITH MUSHROOM CREAM

191 RICE VERMICELLI WITH PRAWNS AND VEGETABLES

193 POLENTA WITH TOMATO SAUCE AND MUSHROOMS

195 LENTIL PASTA WITH TOMATOES AND BASIL

197 SQUID INK RISOTTO WITH PRAWNS

199 KAMUT CAPELLINI WITH GARLIC, OIL AND CHILI PEPPER

201 WHOLE BUTTERFLIES WITH SPINACH AND WALNUT PESTO

203 QUINOA AND BEAN MINESTRONE

205 BUCKWHEAT SPAGHETTI WITH VEGETABLE SAUCE

207 PUMPKIN RAVIOLI WITH BUTTER AND SAGE

209 BARLEY AND VEGETABLE SOUP

211 CHICKPEA LINGUINE WITH TOMATOES AND BLACK OLIVES

RECIPES SECOND DISHES

214 LEMON CHICKEN BREAST WITH BROCCOLETTI

216 GRILLED SALMON WITH AVOCADO SAUCE

218 VEAL PIZZAIOLA WITH TOMATOES AND OREGANO

220 BAKED TROUT FILLET WITH ALMONDS

222 CHICKEN WITH HERBS WITH ASPARAGUS SIDE

224 GRILLED CHICKEN WITH MEDITERRANEAN VEGETABLES

226 TURKEY CURRY WITH VEGETABLES

228 OMELETTE WITH SPINACH AND LOW-HEATER CHEESE

230 STEAMED ASPARAGUS WITH LEMON AND ALMOND SAUCE

232 ROSEMARY CHICKEN WITH COURGETTE SIDE

234 CHICKEN CUTLET WITH ALMONDS AND LINSEED

236 GRILLED TUNA WITH LEMON SAUCE

238 BAKED SALMON WITH LEMON SAUCE AND HERBS

240 TURKEY MEATBALLS WITH CURRY

242 VEAL CHOPS WITH GREEN PEPPER SAUCE

244 SOLE MUGNAIA STYLE WITH CAPERS AND LEMON

246 ROMAN-STYLE ARTICHOKES

248 HERBS BEEF WITH ARUGULA AND TOMATO SALAD

250 GRILLED PRAWNS WITH GARLIC AND PARSLEY SAUCE

252 FISH FRITTERS WITH YOGURT SAUCE

254 AUBERGINES STUFFED WITH QUINOA AND VEGETABLES

256 BEEF STEAK WITH BLACK PEPPER AND TOMATOES

258 VEGETABLE OMELETTE

260 SHRIMP AND VEGETABLES SKEWERS

262 TURKEY SCALOPPINE WITH LEMON AND SAGE

264 CHICKEN SAUSAGES WITH PEPPERS AND ONIONS

266 BAKED TROUT FILLET WITH AROMATIC HERBS

268 GRILLED CHICKEN WITH TOMATO AND BASIL SALAD

270 BAKED COD FILLET WITH OLIVES AND TOMATOES

272 CHICKEN WITH BLACK PEPPER SAUCE AND BROCCOLI SIDE SIDE

SIDE DISH RECIPES

275 SPINACH AND AVOCADO SALAD

277 OVEN GRILLED VEGETABLES

279 BAKED CAULIFLOWER WITH TURMERIC

281 STEAMED BROCCOLI WITH ALMONDS

283 LENTIL SALAD

285 OVEN STUFFED COURGETTES

287 CAULIFLOWER PUREE

289 QUINOA AND VEGETABLES SALAD

291 SAUTEED BLACK CABBAGE WITH GARLIC AND LEMON

293 ROASTED CARROTS WITH THYME

INTRODUCTION TO THE LOW GLYCEMIC INDEX DIET

UNDERSTANDING THE GLYCEMIC INDEX (GI)

In today's nutritional landscape, the low glycemic index (BI) diet stands out as a dietary approach that is gaining more and more attention, offering a path towards overall and lasting well-being.

Based on the principle of regulating the absorption of sugars in the blood, this dietary model is proposed as a simple and versatile strategy to improve health and quality of life. In this introduction, we'll explore the basics of the low glycemic index diet, dispel some common myths, and reveal the secrets to successfully incorporating it into your daily routine. What is the glycemic index (GI)? The glycemic index represents a system of classifying foods based on their ability to influence blood sugar (glycemia) levels after consumption.

Foods are divided into three categories:

High glycemic index (high GI): They cause a rapid increase in blood sugar, followed by an equally rapid drop, with negative effects on blood sugar control and feelings of satiety.

Medium glycemic index (medium GI): They cause a more gradual increase in blood sugar than high GI foods, providing energy more constantly.

Low glycemic index (low GI): They determine a gradual and prolonged increase in blood sugar levels, promoting a lasting sense of satiety and better blood sugar control.

Why follow a low glycemic index diet?

Numerous scientific studies demonstrate that the low glycemic index diet brings numerous health benefits: Optimal blood sugar control: Ideal for people with diabetes or prediabetes, helps stabilize blood sugar levels and reduce the need for medications.

Healthy body weight: Promotes weight loss or maintenance of an ideal body weight, increasing the sense of satiety and reducing hunger pangs.

Cholesterol under control: It can help improve the lipid profile, lowering LDL ("bad") cholesterol levels and increasing HDL ("good") cholesterol.

Reduced risk of heart disease: Reduces the risk of developing cardiovascular disease, thanks to improved blood sugar control and cholesterol levels. **Constant energy during the day:** Provides a constant release of energy, counteracting tiredness and drops in concentration. **Improved Overall Wellbeing:** Promotes a sense of overall well-being, improving mood, sleep quality and digestion.

How to get started with the low glycemic index diet?

Incorporating the low glycemic index diet into your daily routine is simple and enjoyable:

Choose whole foods: Choose whole, unrefined foods, rich in fiber and nutrients. Combine nutrients: Pair low-glycemic foods with protein and healthy fats for a more balanced, filling meal. Limit added sugars: Reduce consumption of sugary drinks, sweets and packaged foods high in added sugars. Cook with healthy methods: Choose steamed, baked or grilled cooking, avoiding fried foods and processed foods. Split meals: Eat 3 main meals and 2-3 snacks during the day to keep blood sugar levels stable. Drink plenty of water: Stay hydrated by drinking water throughout the day to aid satiety and digestion. Consult a professional: A nutritionist or dietician can help you create a personalized meal plan suited to your specific needs. The low glycemic index diet is not just a diet, but a real lifestyle that embraces well-being at 360 degrees. Start your journey to a healthier, more energized future with the low glycemic index diet!

IMPORTANCE OF THE GLYCEMIC INDEX IN THE DIET

The glycemic index (GI) plays a significant role in diet and nutrition for several reasons: 1. Blood sugar control: The GI measures how quickly carbohydrates in foods raise blood glucose levels. Low GI foods cause a gradual and steady rise in blood sugar levels, while high GI foods cause rapid spikes followed by crashes. For people with diabetes or at risk of developing diabetes, understanding GI can help you manage your blood sugar levels more effectively. 2. Satiety and appetite control: Low glycemic index foods are often more filling and provide longer-lasting energy than high glycemic index foods. Eating foods with a lower GI can help control appetite, reduce cravings, and prevent overeating, which is beneficial for weight management and overall health.

3. Energy Levels: Choosing low-glycemic index foods can help maintain stable energy levels throughout the day. Instead of experiencing energy crashes and fatigue after consuming high-glycemic foods, individuals can enjoy sustained energy levels, increased focus, and increased productivity. 4. Weight Management: Including low-glycemic foods in your diet can support weight management efforts. These foods help regulate appetite, reduce calorie intake, and promote fat loss, making them valuable components of a balanced, sustainable weight loss plan. 5. Heart Health: High glycemic index diets have been associated with an increased risk of cardiovascular disease.

On the other hand, diets rich in low-glycemic index foods, such as whole grains, fruits, vegetables and legumes, can help lower cholesterol levels, improve blood lipid profiles and reduce the risk of heart disease. 6. Diabetes Management and Prevention: For people with diabetes, understanding and incorporating low-glycemic foods into your diet can help stabilize blood sugar levels, reduce insulin resistance, and decrease the need for insulin medications. Additionally, adopting a low glycemic index diet can help prevent the onset of type 2 diabetes in high-risk individuals. 7. General health and well-being: Consuming a diet rich in low-glycemic index foods can contribute to overall health and well-being by providing essential nutrients, fiber, vitamins and minerals.

These foods support digestive health, immune function and optimal metabolic function, promoting longevity and vitality. In conclusion, the glycemic index is an essential tool for making informed dietary choices that support blood sugar control, weight management, heart health and overall well-being. By incorporating low-GI foods into the diet and minimizing high-GI foods, individuals can optimize their health and reduce the risk of chronic disease.

BASICS OF THE GLYCEMIC INDEX

WHAT IS THE GLYCEMIC INDEX

The glycemic index (GI) is a measurement used to evaluate how quickly carbohydrates found in different foods raise blood sugar levels after consumption compared to pure glucose, which has a GI value of 100. Here are the basics glycemic index: 1. Scale: The GI scale ranges from 0 to 100, with pure glucose having a GI value of 100. Foods are classified into three categories based on their GI value: Low GI: 55 or less Medium GI: 56/69 High GI: 70 or higher 2. Impact on blood sugar: Foods with a high GI cause a rapid rise in blood sugar levels, while those with a low GI cause a slower rise and gradual. This is important for people managing diabetes, as it helps them choose foods that help keep blood sugar levels stable.

3. Factors Affecting GI: Several factors influence the GI of a food, including the type of carbohydrate, fiber content, fat and protein content, food processing, and cooking methods. Generally, foods with more fiber, fat and protein tend to have a lower GI. **4. Low-GI foods:** Examples of low-GI foods include most non-starchy vegetables, legumes (beans, lentils), whole grains (barley, quinoa, oats), fruits (apples, berries, citrus fruits).) and dairy products. **5. High-glycemic foods:** High-glycemic foods include refined grains (white bread, white rice, sugary cereals), potatoes, sugary snacks and desserts, and sugary drinks. **6. Glycemic Load (CG):** The glycemic load takes into account both the GI of a food and the size of the portion consumed. It provides a more accurate measure of how a particular food affects blood sugar levels.

Low GL foods have minimal impact on blood sugar levels. 7. Practical Application: Understanding the GI of foods can help people make healthier food choices. Opting for low-glycemic foods can help manage hunger, control blood sugar levels and reduce the risk of chronic diseases such as type 2 diabetes and heart disease. In summary, the glycemic index is a valuable tool for understanding how different carbohydrates affect blood sugar levels. By focusing on consuming low-GI foods and moderating high-GI foods, individuals can make informed choices to support their overall health and well-being.

HOW FOODS AFFECT BLOOD SUGAR LEVELS

The glycemic index (GI) is a system that ranks carbohydrates in foods based on how they affect blood sugar levels after consumption. It measures how quickly carbohydrates are broken down and absorbed into the bloodstream, leading to increased blood glucose (sugar) levels. Here's how the glycemic index works: 1. Scoring system: The glycemic index assigns a numerical value to different carbohydrate-containing foods, typically between 0 and 100. Pure glucose is used as a reference point and has a GI value of 100, which represents the highest possible glycemic response. 2. Categories: Foods are classified into three main groups based on glycemic index values: low GI (55 or lower) medium GI (56 to 69) high GI (70 or higher)

3. Impact on blood sugar: Foods with a high glycemic index cause a rapid spike in blood sugar levels after consumption, followed by a rapid decline. These foods include white bread, white rice, sugary snacks, and most processed foods. 4. Slow release of glucose: In contrast, foods with a low glycemic index lead to a slower and more gradual increase in blood sugar levels. These foods are typically higher in fiber, protein and healthy fats and include whole grains, legumes, fruits and vegetables. 5. Factors that influence GI: Several factors can influence the glycemic index of a food, including: Type of carbohydrate: Simple carbohydrates are usually digested more quickly than complex carbohydrates. Fiber content: Fiber-rich foods tend to have a lower glycemic index because fiber slows the digestion and absorption of carbohydrates. Processing and cooking methods:

Processing and cooking can affect the GI of foods. For example, overcooking pasta can increase its GI. 6. Practical Applications: Understanding the glycemic index can be helpful in managing blood sugar levels, especially for people with diabetes. By choosing foods with a lower glycemic index, they can help stabilize blood sugar levels and reduce the risk of insulin resistance and type 2 diabetes. In summary, the glycemic index provides information on how different carbohydrates affect sugar levels in the blood. It serves as a helpful tool for making informed dietary choices that support overall health and well-being, especially for people concerned about blood sugar regulation.

HEALTH IMPACTS

IMPACT ON WEIGHT MANAGEMENT

Foods influence weight management in various ways, and their impact depends on the nutritional composition and quantity consumed. Here's how different types of foods can affect weight management: 1. High in Fiber and Low Glycemic Index: Foods high in fiber and with a low glycemic index tend to be more filling and provide energy more gradually. This can help control appetite and reduce the risk of overeating, contributing to weight loss and maintaining a healthy weight. 2. High in Protein: Foods rich in protein, such as lean meat, fish, eggs, low-fat dairy products, legumes and tofu, can promote satiety and help preserve muscle mass during weight loss. Proteins also require more energy to digest than carbohydrates and fats.

3. Healthy Fats: Mono- and polyunsaturated fatty acids, found in foods such as avocados, nuts, seeds, vegetable oils and fatty fish, can contribute to a feeling of satiety and support cardiometabolic health. However, it is important to consume them in moderation as they are caloric. 4. Processed and High-Sugar Foods: Processed foods, rich in added sugars, saturated fats and salt, are often calorie-dense and less filling. Excessive consumption of such foods can contribute to weight gain and increase the risk of obesity and related diseases. 5. Portions and Calorie Control: Regardless of nutritional composition, consuming excessive portions of food can lead to excess calories and weight gain. Portion control and awareness of calorie intake are crucial to maintaining or losing weight healthily.

6. Energy Balance: Weight management depends on energy balance, i.e. the ratio between calories consumed through food and calories burned through physical activity and basal metabolism. To lose weight, you need to create a calorie deficit by consuming fewer calories than you burn, while maintaining weight requires a balance between calorie intake and consumption. In conclusion, a balanced and varied diet rich in whole foods, fruits, vegetables, lean proteins and healthy fats, combined with portion control and an active lifestyle, can support weight management effectively and healthily. It is important to adopt long-term sustainable eating habits and consult a health professional for personalized support in weight management.

GLYCEMIC INDEX AND METABOLIC HEALTH

The Glycemic Index (GI) plays a significant role in metabolic health, influencing several aspects of glucose and insulin metabolism in the body. Here's how the Glycemic Index can influence metabolic health: 1. Blood Glucose Control: The Glycemic Index measures how quickly carbohydrates in foods raise blood sugar levels. Foods with a low GI cause a more gradual and controlled increase in blood sugar, while those with a high GI cause more rapid and pronounced blood sugar spikes. Maintaining stable blood glucose levels is critical to metabolic health, especially for individuals with diabetes or at risk of developing it.

2. Insulin Sensitivity: Consuming foods with a low Glycemic Index can improve insulin sensitivity, which means that the body's cells respond better to the insulin produced by the pancreas. Increased insulin sensitivity reduces the risk of developing insulin resistance and type 2 diabetes. **3. Weight Management:** Choosing foods with a low GI can promote weight loss and maintenance of a healthy body weight. Low GI foods tend to be more satiating and provide a more stable source of energy throughout the day, reducing the risk of overeating and unhealthy snacking. **4. Appetite Control:** Low GI foods help control appetite and food cravings, as they provide a longer-lasting feeling of satiety than high GI foods. This can contribute to better management of overall calorie intake and prevention of obesity.

5. Cardiovascular Health: Consuming foods with a low GI can improve cardiovascular risk factors, such as LDL ("bad") cholesterol and blood triglyceride levels. This can reduce the risk of heart disease and stroke. 6. Energy Control: Low GI foods provide a more consistent release of energy throughout the day, avoiding sudden spikes and dips in energy. This can improve mood, concentration and cognitive performance. In summary, adopting a diet based on foods with a low Glycemic Index can have numerous benefits for metabolic health, helping to maintain stable blood glucose levels, improve insulin sensitivity, promote weight loss and reduce the risk of chronic diseases. Incorporating a variety of whole foods, fruits, vegetables, legumes and lean proteins can help optimize metabolic and overall health.

IMPLEMENTATION OF THE GLYCEMIC INDEX DIET

CHOOSE FOODS WITH A LOW GLYCEMIC INDEX

It's an important step in keeping blood sugar levels stable and promoting good metabolic health. Here are some examples of low glycemic index foods to include in your diet: 1. Non-starchy vegetables: Spinach, broccoli, cauliflower, carrots, zucchini, tomatoes, peppers, cucumbers, lettuce, asparagus, arugula. 2. Fresh fruit: Apples, pears, strawberries, blueberries, raspberries, peaches, apricots, oranges, kiwis, plums, cherries. 3. Whole grains: Quinoa, spelt, bulgur, barley, buckwheat, brown rice, oats, whole grains. 4. Legumes: Lentils, black beans, cannellini beans, chickpeas, peas, red beans, borlotti beans.

5. Lean protein: Skinless chicken, turkey, fish (salmon, tuna, trout, sole), eggs, tofu, tempeh. **6. Nuts and seeds:** Almonds, walnuts, hazelnuts, chia seeds, flax seeds, sunflower seeds, pumpkin seeds. **7. Low-fat dairy products:** Natural Greek yogurt, skim or low-fat milk, low-fat cream cheese. **8. Healthy graphs:** Extra virgin olive oil, coconut oil, flaxseed oil, avocado, nuts, seeds. **9. Spices and aromatic herbs:** Turmeric, ginger, black pepper, parsley, basil, oregano, rosemary, thyme. **10. Whole grain foods:**

Wholemeal bread, wholemeal pasta, brown rice, spelt, buckwheat, bulgur. Including a variety of these foods in your daily diet can help keep blood sugar levels stable, promote a feeling of satiety, and provide essential nutrients for overall good health. Remember to combine foods in a balanced way and pay attention to portions to get the maximum benefit from your diet.

CREATE BALANCED MEALS

involves combining a variety of foods that provide all the essential nutrients the body needs to function optimally. Here are some tips for creating balanced meals: 1. Include a source of protein: Lean meat (chicken, turkey, fish), eggs, low-fat dairy (Greek yogurt, skim milk), legumes (lentils, beans, chickpeas) , tofu or tempeh. 2. Add complex carbohydrates: Whole grains (brown rice, quinoa, spelt, barley), wholemeal bread, wholemeal pasta, sweet potatoes, legumes, starchy vegetables (potatoes, corn, peas). 3. Incorporate a variety of vegetables: Dark leafy greens (spinach, kale, arugula), cruciferous vegetables (broccoli, cauliflower, cabbage), carrots, peppers, tomatoes, cucumbers, zucchini, eggplant, etc.

4. Add healthy fats: Avocado, unrefined vegetable oils (extra virgin olive oil, coconut oil), nuts, seeds, nut butters, fatty fish (salmon, sardines). 5. Includes sources of fiber: Whole grains, legumes, vegetables, fresh fruit with peel, nuts and seeds. 6. Limit added sugars and processed foods: Reduce your consumption of foods high in added sugars, such as sweets, sugary drinks, packaged snacks and processed foods. 7. Balance your portions: Keep portions of each food group balanced. For example, half of your plate can be made up of vegetables, a quarter of protein and a quarter of complex carbohydrates. 8. Hydration: Drink plenty of water throughout the day. Avoid sugary drinks and carbonated drinks.

9. Be careful with culinary preparations: Opt for healthy cooking methods such as steaming, grilling, baking or pan-cooking rather than frying or cooking with excess added fat. 10. Plan ahead: Prepare meals ahead of time whenever possible to avoid unhealthy food choices throughout the day. By following these tips, you can create balanced meals that provide your body with the energy and nutrients it needs to function at its best. Remember to listen to your body and tailor portions and food choices to your individual needs and health goals.

MEAL PLANNING STRATEGIES

Meal planning is an effective strategy for adopting healthy eating habits and better managing your time and cooking resources. Here are some meal planning strategies that can help you: 1. Set a fixed day for meal planning: Choose a fixed day of the week to plan the next week's meals. This will allow you to organize yourself better and shop based on the necessary ingredients. 2. Create a weekly menu: Prepare a weekly menu that includes breakfasts, lunches, dinners and snacks. Be sure to include a variety of foods and dishes to balance the diet. 3. Consider needs and preferences: Take your family's dietary needs, food preferences and busy schedules into account when planning meals. Try to include foods that everyone enjoys and that meet the nutritional needs of all family members.

4. Make use of leftovers: Plan meals so you can use leftover ingredients already in the fridge and pantry. This will reduce waste and help you save time and money. **5. Batch prepare meals:** Make extra portions of foods that keep well and can be eaten multiple times throughout the week, such as soups, stews, chili, salads, etc. **6. Make a shopping list:** Once you have planned your meals, create a detailed shopping list with all the necessary ingredients. This way you will avoid forgetting something and buying unnecessary foods. **7. Choose quick and simple recipes:** Opt for quick and simple recipes during the busiest days of the week. You can save time by preparing meals that require few ingredients and little prep time.

8. Variety and Balance: Be sure to include a variety of foods and nutrients in your planned meals, balancing proteins, complex carbohydrates, healthy fats, fiber, vitamins and minerals. 9. Flexibility: Be flexible with meal planning and adapt the menu according to unexpected events and changes in the agenda. 10. Prepare ahead of time: Whenever possible, prep ingredients ahead of time or prepare main meals ahead of time and store them in the refrigerator or freezer for quick access throughout the week. Meal planning takes some time and organization up front, but it can make nutrition management more efficient and support healthier, more balanced food choices in the long term.

PRACTICAL TIPS FOR SUCCESS

BUY FOODS WITH A LOW GLYCEMIC INDEX

Buying low-glycemic foods can be a helpful strategy for promoting metabolic health and keeping blood sugar levels stable. Here are some tips on how to select low-GI foods while shopping: 1. Prefer whole grains: Choose whole-wheat bread, whole-wheat pasta, brown rice, quinoa, spelt and other whole grains over their refined high-GI counterparts. 2. Opt for legumes: Buy a variety of legumes such as lentils, beans, chickpeas and peas.

3. Include plenty of veggies: Fill your grocery cart with a variety of fresh veggies, including broccoli, spinach, cabbage, carrots, zucchini, tomatoes and peppers. Non-starchy vegetables are generally low-glycemic and rich in fiber and nutrients. 4. Choose fresh fruit: Opt for low-glycemic fresh fruit such as apples, pears, strawberries, blueberries, raspberries, cherries, oranges and kiwis. Avoid fruit varieties that are too ripe or too sugary. 5. Read food labels: Check food labels for products with low added sugars and refined ingredients. Avoid packaged foods and snacks that are high in sugar and refined carbohydrates. 6. Limit processed foods: Minimize your consumption of processed foods such as cookies, sweets, snacks and packaged foods, which often contain added sugars and other high-glycemic ingredients.

7. Buy lean protein sources: Choose lean meats like chicken, turkey, fish and eggs, as well as low-fat dairy products like Greek yogurt and low-fat cheese. 8. Supplement with healthy fats: Buy healthy fats like avocados, nuts, seeds, extra virgin olive oil and coconut oil to add flavor and nutrients to meals. 9. Plan carefully: Make a shopping list based on the meals you have planned for the week to avoid impulse purchases and keep the focus on low-glycemic index foods. 10. Make conscious choices: Choosing low-GI foods isn't about limiting yourself to a few foods, but rather expanding the variety and balance in your diet to promote metabolic health and overall well-being.

TIPS FOR COOKING AND PREPARING FOOD

Here are some useful tips for cooking and preparing food in a healthy and tasty way: 1. Use light cooking methods: Prefer light cooking methods such as steaming, grilling, baking, cooking in a non-stick pan or cooking baked in foil. These methods reduce the use of added fats and preserve the natural flavor of foods. 2. Limit the use of saturated fats: Reduce the use of saturated fats such as butter and margarine and prefer healthy fats such as extra virgin olive oil, coconut oil, sunflower oil and flaxseed oil. 3. Experiment with herbs and spices: Use a variety of fresh herbs and spices to add flavor to your dishes without adding salt or high-sodium seasonings. Try basil, parsley, oregano, rosemary, thyme, black pepper, turmeric, ginger, paprika and cinnamon.

4. Add plenty of veggies: Increase the amount of veggies in your dishes by adding a variety of colors and flavors. Vegetables not only add fiber and essential nutrients, but they also help make meals more filling and filling. **5. Choose fresh, seasonal ingredients:** Go for fresh, seasonal and local ingredients whenever possible. Fresh ingredients offer the best flavor and nutritional value. **6. Reduce the use of added sugars:** Limit the use of added sugars in your dishes. Use natural sugar alternatives like honey, maple syrup or stevia to sweeten recipes. **7. Balance flavors:** Experiment with a variety of contrasting and complementary flavors in your dishes. Balance sweet with bitter, sour with sweet, and spicy with creamy to create balanced and satisfying dishes.

8. Batch prepare meals: Spend time preparing batch meals on the weekend or when you have more time on your hands. You can cook large quantities of food and store them to have meals ready to reheat throughout the week. **9. Be creative:** Experiment with new recipes, ingredients and flavor combinations to make cooking a fun and inspiring experience. **10. Enjoy the process:** Preparing food can be a relaxing and satisfying time. Take advantage of the time spent in the kitchen to connect with food and with those who will share it with you. By following these tips, you can prepare delicious, nutritious meals that will contribute to your well-being and that of your loved ones.

EATING OUT WHILE FOLLOWING A LOW GLYCEMIC DIET

Eating out while on a low-glycemic diet can be a challenge, but you can make conscious food choices to keep your blood sugar levels stable. Here are some tips for eating out on a glycemic index: 1. Choose restaurants with healthy options: Look for restaurants that offer healthy, balanced menu options, such as fresh salads, fish or lean meat dishes, and vegetable sides. 2. Read the menu carefully: Before ordering, take time to read the menu carefully and look for dishes featuring lean proteins, complex carbohydrates and vegetables. Avoid fried dishes, sandwiches and foods high in added sugars.

3. Ask questions to the staff: Don't hesitate to ask questions to the restaurant staff about the ingredients and preparation methods of the dishes. Ask if you can make changes to the dish to make it more suitable for your low-glycemic diet. **4. Choose moderate portions:** Try to avoid excessively large portions and try to keep portions moderate. If the plate is too large, consider splitting the portion or taking the leftovers home for a later meal. **5. Avoid sugary drinks:** Limit the consumption of sugary drinks such as sodas, fruit juices and sweet cocktails. Opt for water, unsweetened teas or herbal drinks to reduce your added sugar intake. **6. Be careful with sauces and conditions:** Many sauces and condiments may contain added sugars and refined carbohydrates. Choose light sauces or ask to have the sauces served on the side so you can control the amount you use.

7. Order appetizers and sides: If you don't find main options that fit your diet, consider ordering a variety of appetizers or sides that follow the principles of the low-glycemic index diet. 8. Be aware of food combinations: Try to balance meals with a combination of proteins, complex carbohydrates and healthy fats to keep blood sugar levels stable and promote a feeling of satiety. 9. Avoid foods rich in simple carbohydrates: Limit consumption of high glycemic index foods such as white bread, white rice, French fries and sweets high in sugar. 10. Enjoy your meal: Eating out should be an enjoyable experience. Try to focus on enjoying the meal and the company rather than the stress of choosing foods. With a little planning and awareness, you can maintain a low glycemic index diet even when eating out.

MANAGE CHALLENGES OVERCOMING COMMON OBSTACLES

Overcoming common obstacles related to diet and maintaining a healthy lifestyle can require commitment and awareness. Here are some tips for addressing some common challenges: 1. Lack of time: Organize your time to include meal preparation and physical activity in your daily routine. Plan your meals for the week in advance and look for quick, healthy recipes that fit your lifestyle. 2. Socialization and external pressures: Communicate openly with friends and family about your health goals so they can support you. Choose restaurants that offer healthy options and make conscious choices when invited to social events.

3. Stress and emotionality: Find healthy ways to manage stress, such as meditation, yoga, physical activity or therapy. Try to identify your emotional triggers and develop alternative strategies to deal with them without resorting to food. 4. Satiety and hunger: Maintain satiety by choosing foods rich in fiber, protein and healthy fats that help you feel full longer. Avoid letting yourself get hungry and plan healthy snacks to avoid overindulging during main meals. 5. Lacks motivation: Find a personal, meaningful reason to adopt a healthy lifestyle. It could be improving health, increasing energy, or achieving a specific goal. Keep motivation alive with small successes and non-food rewards. 6. Lack of knowledge: Educate yourself about healthy food options and learn to read food labels to make informed choices.

Consult a health professional, such as a nutritionist or dietician, for personalized advice and support. 7. Relapses and mistakes: Accept that relapses can happen and that they are part of the journey of self-improvement. Don't punish yourself for mistakes, but learn from them and get back to your healthy routine right away. 8. Resistance to change: Make small, incremental changes rather than trying to radically transform your life overnight. Be kind to yourself and recognize your successes, even the small ones. Tackling these obstacles takes time, patience, and consistent effort, but with determination and proper support, you can overcome them and achieve your long-term health goals.

ADAPT YOUR DIET TO DIFFERENT LIFESTYLES

Adapting your diet to different lifestyles is essential to ensure it is sustainable and in line with individual needs. Here are some tips for adapting your diet to various lifestyles: 1. Active lifestyle: If you are an active person or regularly engage in physical activity, make sure you include enough complex carbohydrates in your diet to provide energy and support your physical activity . Lean proteins and healthy fats should be an integral part of your meals for muscle repair and recovery. 2. Sedentary lifestyle: If you lead a more sedentary lifestyle, be sure to carefully monitor the amount of calories you eat and be careful not to overindulge in large portions. Focus on whole foods, fiber and nutrient dense foods to maintain metabolic health and manage weight.

3. Demanding Work: If you have a job that requires physical or mental exertion, be sure to plan meals that give you the energy and focus you need throughout the day. Opt for balanced meals that include proteins, complex carbohydrates and healthy fats. 4. Frequent Travel: If you travel frequently for work or pleasure, plan your meals in advance and look for healthy options at restaurants or airports. Bring along healthy snacks such as dried fruit, homemade protein bars or cut vegetables to avoid having to make unhealthy food choices in case of sudden hunger. 5. Irregular Schedules: If your meal times are irregular due to work or other commitments, try to maintain consistency in your food choices.

Stock up on healthy foods that can be consumed quickly when you're on the go, and plan balanced meals when you have more time on your hands.

6. Budget Constraints: If you have budget constraints, plan inexpensive but nutritious meals using inexpensive ingredients like legumes, whole grains, seasonal vegetables, and lean proteins like eggs and chicken. 7. Vegetarian or Vegan Diet: If you follow a vegetarian or vegan diet, make sure you get enough protein from plant sources like legumes, tofu, tempeh, quinoa, and seeds. Be careful to supplement your diet with essential vitamins and minerals such as vitamin B12, iron and calcium. 8. Food intolerances or allergies: If you have food intolerances or allergies, adapt your diet by avoiding foods that trigger an allergic reaction or digestive discomfort.

Look for nutritious and tasty alternatives to replace the foods you need to eliminate from your diet. Furthermore, it is important to be flexible and adapt your diet according to your personal needs and preferences. Listen to your body and make adjustments when necessary to ensure your nutrition supports your lifestyle and overall well-being.

4. Find support: Seek support from friends, family or support groups who share your health goals. Sharing challenges and successes with others can make the journey more manageable and motivating. 5. Make wellness a priority: Remember that taking care of yourself is important. Set aside time every day to exercise, relax, sleep well and nourish your body with nutritious foods. 6. Visualize your success: Imagine yourself achieving your health goals. Visualize how you will feel and what you will do when you reach your goals.

This can help you stay motivated and focused on your path. 7. Be flexible: Life is full of unexpected events and obstacles. Be flexible in your approaches and adapt your strategy when necessary. Don't be afraid to make changes to your plan if it isn't working as expected.

8. Remember your "why": Always keep in mind why you started this journey to a healthier life. This "why" can give you the motivation you need to overcome challenges and continue to progress. With determination, commitment, and a positive mindset, you are on the right path to continued success in your glycemic index diet and your path to better overall health and well-being.

ADDITIONAL INFORMATION ON THE GLYCEMIC INDEX

Here is some additional information about the glycemic index (GI) that may be helpful: 1. Glycemic Index Definition: The Glycemic Index is a scale that measures how quickly a carbohydrate-containing food raises blood glucose levels relative to a food reference, usually glucose or white bread. Foods are classified according to their GI as low, medium or high. 2. Factors that influence the Glycemic Index: Various factors can influence the GI of a food, including chemical composition, presence of fiber, food handling and cooking, combination of foods in a meal, and maturation of fruits. 3. High GI Foods: High GI foods cause a rapid increase in blood sugar levels.

These include foods such as white bread, sweets, sugary drinks, chips, and refined grains. 4. Low GI Foods: Low GI foods produce a gradual increase in blood sugar levels. These include non-starchy fruits and vegetables, legumes, whole grains, low-fat dairy products, and some sources of protein. 5. Importance of the Glycemic Index in the Diet: Managing the GI of the foods consumed can be useful for controlling blood sugar levels, maintaining the feeling of satiety for longer, reducing the risk of developing type 2 diabetes and helping in weight loss. 6. Postprandial Blood Sugar: Postprandial blood sugar is the blood sugar level after a meal. Reducing the GI of foods consumed can help keep postprandial blood sugar within acceptable limits, which is important for metabolic health and chronic disease prevention.

7. Meal Planning: Planning meals considering the GI of foods can help create more balanced and healthy meals. Combining low GI foods with lean proteins, healthy fats and fiber can help keep blood sugar levels stable and promote better overall health. 8. Monitoring the Glycemic Index: You can find tables and databases online that provide information on the GI of foods. These resources can be helpful in planning meals and making more informed food choices. Understanding the GI of foods and how it affects metabolic health can be an important component of a balanced and healthy diet. Incorporating low GI foods into your daily diet can help improve overall well-being and prevent conditions related to high blood sugar.

WHAT IS THE GLYCEMIC INDEX DIET

The Glycemic Index Diet is a dietary approach that is based on the concept of the glycemic index (GI). The glycemic index measures how quickly a food raises blood sugar levels after being consumed. Foods with a high glycemic index cause a rapid increase in blood sugar, while those with a low glycemic index cause a more gradual and controlled increase in blood sugar. The goal of the glycemic index diet is to choose foods with a lower GI to stabilize blood sugar levels, control appetite and promote greater feelings of satiety. Additionally, this diet can help improve insulin sensitivity and manage body weight.

Low-GI foods include non-starchy vegetables, legumes, whole grains, fresh fruit, low-fat dairy products and lean proteins. In contrast, high glycemic index foods include refined sugars, white bread, white rice, potatoes and sweet snacks. The Glycemic Index Diet encourages the consumption of whole, unprocessed foods, promoting a diet rich in fiber, vitamins and minerals. Furthermore, it promotes portion control and overall diet balance. This dietary approach may be especially helpful for people with type 2 diabetes, as it can help improve glycemic control. However, it is important to consult a health professional before adopting any diet, especially if you have pre-existing medical conditions.

THE BENEFITS OF THE DIET

The Glycemic Index Diet offers several health benefits: 1. Weight control: Low glycemic index foods tend to produce a longer-lasting feeling of satiety, thus reducing hunger and the desire for unhealthy snacks between meals. This can help with weight control and appetite management. 2. Stabilization of blood sugar levels: Adopting a low glycemic index diet can help keep blood sugar levels more stable throughout the day, reducing the risk of glycemic spikes and reactive hypoglycemia. 3. Better insulin control: A low glycemic index diet can improve insulin sensitivity and reduce insulin resistance, thereby helping to prevent or manage type 2 diabetes.

4. Promote cardiometabolic health: By reducing consumption of high-glycemic foods, the diet can help improve blood cholesterol levels, reducing the risk of cardiovascular disease and improving overall heart health. 5. Better energy management: Low glycemic index foods provide a more stable and long-lasting source of energy than high glycemic index foods, helping to maintain a constant level of energy throughout the day. 6. Promote a balanced diet: The glycemic index diet promotes the consumption of whole foods, fruits, vegetables, whole grains and lean proteins, thus encouraging a balanced, nutrient-rich diet. 7. Appetite Control: Low glycemic index foods tend to be more filling, which can help reduce the overall amount of food consumed and prevent overeating.

8. Improved digestive health: Low glycemic index foods are often rich in fiber, which can support digestive health, improve bowel regularity and reduce the risk of digestive diseases. Adopting the Glycemic Index Diet can help improve general health and prevent a series of pathologies related to diet and lifestyle. However, it is important to remember that a balanced diet and healthy lifestyle are key to achieving maximum health benefits.

RECIPES APPETIZERS

WHOLE WHOLE BRUSCHETTA WITH TOMATOES AND FRESH BASIL

Preparation time: 10 minutes

Cooking times: 5 minutes

Doses for 4 people:

Ingredients

Wholemeal bread: 400g

Cherry tomatoes: 250g

Fresh basil: 30g

Garlic: 2 cloves

Extra virgin olive oil: 60ml

Salt and Pepper To Taste

Preparation:

Cut the wholemeal bread into slices and grill it lightly. Cut the cherry tomatoes in half and chop the fresh basil. Peel the garlic cloves and rub them on the slices of grilled bread. Distribute the cherry tomatoes and basil on the bread slices. Season with extra virgin olive oil, salt and pepper. Serve immediately. Nutritional values (per serving): Calories: 220 kcal Proteins: 6g Fat: 8g Carbohydrates: 30g Fibre: 5g Sugars: 4g Sodium: 300mg.

WHOLE BREAD CROUTTONS WITH BLACK OLIVE PÂTÉ

Preparation time: 15 minutes

Cooking times: 0 minutes

Doses for 4 people:

Ingredients:

Wholemeal bread: 300g

Pitted black olives: 150g

Anchovies in oil: 50g

Capers: 30g

Extra virgin olive oil: 60ml

Lemon juice: 1 tbsp

Ground black pepper to taste

Preparation:

Cut the wholemeal bread into slices and toast them lightly. In the blender, combine the black olives, anchovies, capers, extra virgin olive oil and lemon juice. Blend until you obtain a creamy consistency. Spread the paté obtained on the slices of toasted bread. Add ground black pepper to taste. Serve as an appetizer or snack. These delicious recipes are perfect for a healthy and tasty cooking experience! Nutritional values (per serving): Calories: 180 kcal Proteins: 4g Fat: 10g Carbohydrates: 15g Fibre: 3g Sugars: 1g Sodium: 350mg.

CAPRESE SALAD WITH LIGHT MOZZARELLA AND CHERRY TOMATOES

Preparation time: 10 minutes

Cooking times: 0 minutes

Doses for 4 people:

Ingredients

Light mozzarella: 200g

Cherry tomatoes: 300g

Fresh basil: 20g

Extra virgin olive oil: 30ml

Balsamic vinegar: 15ml

Salt and Pepper To Taste

Preparation:

Cut the light mozzarella into thin slices and the cherry tomatoes in half. Arrange the mozzarella slices and cherry tomatoes alternately on a serving plate. Add fresh basil leaves between the layers. Season with extra virgin olive oil, balsamic vinegar, salt and pepper. Serve fresh. 7. Nutritional Values (per approximate portion): Calories: 120 kcal Protein: 8g Fat: 7g Carbohydrates: 5g Fibre: 1g Sugars: 3g Sodium: 250mg

RAW HAM WITH MELON SLICES

Preparation time: 5 minutes

Cooking times: 0 minutes

Doses for 4 people:

Ingredients:

Raw ham: 150g

Melon: 400g

Preparation:

Cut the melon into slices and remove the seeds. Wrap each slice of melon with a slice of raw ham. Arrange the rolls on a serving plate. Serve fresh. 7. Nutritional Values (per approximate portion): Calories: 90 kcal Protein: 6g Fat: 3g Carbohydrates: 10g Fibre: 1g Sugars: 10g Sodium: 450mg.

CARPACCIO OF COURGETTE WITH SKYNNY CHEESE AND EXTRA VIRGIN OLIVE OIL

Preparation time: 15 minutes

Cooking times: 0 minutes

Doses for 4 people:

Ingredients:

Courgettes: 300g

Sliced low-fat cheese: 150g

Extra virgin olive oil: 30ml

Lemon juice: 15ml

Salt and Pepper To Taste

Preparation:

Cut the courgettes into thin slices with a mandolin or sharp knife. Arrange the courgette slices on a serving plate. Add the low-fat cheese slices on top of the zucchini. Season with extra virgin olive oil, lemon juice, salt and pepper. Serve fresh. Nutritional values: (per serving): Calories: 120 kcal Protein: 8g Fat: 9g Carbohydrates: 4g Fibre: 2g Sugars: 2g Sodium: 250mg.

SEAFOOD SALAD WITH SHRIMPS AND AVOCADO

Preparation time: 10 minutes

Cooking times: 5 minutes

(for cooking shrimp)

Doses for 4 people:

Ingredients:

Shelled shrimp: 250g

Ripe avocado: 2

Mixed lettuce: 200g

Cherry tomatoes: 150g

Lemon juice: 30ml

Extra virgin olive oil: 30ml

Salt and Pepper To Taste

Preparation:

Cook the prawns in boiling salted water for about 3/5 minutes, until they become pink and opaque. Drain them and let them cool. Cut the avocados into cubes and the cherry tomatoes in half. Arrange the mixed lettuce on a serving plate. Add the avocados, cherry tomatoes and shrimp over the lettuce. Season with lemon juice, extra virgin olive oil, salt and pepper. Serve immediately. Be sure to adjust ingredient quantities based on your preferences and dietary needs. Nutritional values: (per serving): Calories: 180 kcal Protein: 10g Fat: 12g Carbohydrates: 10g Fibre: 6g Sugars: 2g Sodium: 350mg.

GRILLED AUBERGINE ROLLS WITH LIGHT RICOTTA

Preparation time: 20 minutes

Cooking times: 15 minutes

Doses for 4 people:

Ingredients:

Aubergines: 2 large (about 400g)

Light ricotta: 200g

Dried tomatoes in oil: 50g

Light grated cheese: 30g

Fresh basil: 20g

Extra virgin olive oil: 30ml

Salt and Pepper To Taste

Preparation:

Slice the aubergines lengthwise, brush them with oil and grill them until soft. In a bowl, mix the ricotta with the chopped dried tomatoes, grated cheese, chopped basil, salt and pepper. Divide the ricotta mixture over the aubergine slices and roll them up. Secure the rolls with toothpicks and grill for a few minutes. Serve hot. Nutritional values (per serving): Calories: 180 kcal Proteins: 8g Fat: 10g Carbohydrates: 15g Fibre: 5g Sugars: 3g Sodium: 300mg

PUMPKIN SOUP WITH ROSEMARY WHOLE CROUTONS

Preparation time: 20 minutes 3.

Cooking times: 30 minutes 4.

Doses for 4 people: 5.

Ingredients:

Pumpkin: 1 kg

Onion: 1 large (about 150g)

Potatoes: 2 medium (about 300g)

Vegetable broth: 1 litre

Extra virgin olive oil: 30ml

Salt and Pepper To Taste

Wholemeal bread: 200g

Fresh rosemary: 10g

Preparation:

Cut the pumpkin, potatoes and onion into coarse pieces. In a pan, fry the onion in olive oil until golden brown, then add the pumpkin and potatoes. Cover with vegetable broth and cook until the vegetables are tender. Blend everything until you obtain a smooth cream, add salt and pepper. For the croutons: cut the bread into slices, brush with olive oil, sprinkle with chopped rosemary and bake in the oven until golden. Serve the cream soup with hot croutons. Be sure to adjust ingredient quantities based on your preferences and dietary needs. Nutritional values (per serving) Calories: 120 kcal Proteins: 3g Fat: 4g Carbohydrates: 20g Fibre: 5g Sugars: 5g Sodium: 300mg.

ZUCCHINI AND CHICKPEA FLOUR FRITTERS

Preparation time: 15 minutes

Cooking times: 10 minutes

Doses for 4 people:

Ingredients:

Zucchini: 400g

Chickpea flour: 150g

Eggs: 2 Chopped onion: 1 small

Chopped fresh parsley: 2 tablespoons

Salt and Pepper To Taste

Extra virgin olive oil

for frying: as needed

Preparation:

Grate the courgettes and squeeze them to remove excess water. In a bowl, mix the grated courgettes with the chickpea flour, eggs, chopped onion, parsley, salt and pepper. Heat some olive oil in a non-stick pan. Form pancakes with the mixture and fry them until golden on both sides. Drain them on absorbent paper to remove excess oil. Serve hot with a sauce of your choice. 7. Nutritional Values (per approximate serving): Calories: 180 kcal Protein: 8g Fat: 7g Carbohydrates: 20g Fibre: 4g Sugars: 3g Sodium: 300mg.

SALMON TARTARE WITH AVOCADO AND LIME

Preparation time: 20 minutes

Cooking times: 0 minutes

Doses for 4 people:

Ingredients:

Fresh salmon: 300g

Ripe avocado: 2

Files: 2

Chopped red onion: 1 small

Chopped fresh parsley: 2 tablespoons

Salt and Pepper To Taste

Extra virgin olive oil: 2 tablespoons

Preparation:

Cut the salmon into small cubes and place it in a bowl. Mash the avocados and add them to the salmon along with the chopped red onion, parsley, lime juice, olive oil, salt and pepper. Mix gently. Shape portions using a pastry cutter and arrange them on serving plates. Decorate with lime slices and parsley leaves, if desired. Serve cold. 7. Nutritional Values (per approximate serving): Calories: 220 kcal Protein: 15g Fat: 12g Carbohydrates: 10g Fibre: 5g Sugars: 2g Sodium: 300mg.

QUINOA SALAD WITH MIXED VEGETABLES

Preparation time: 15 minutes

Cooking times: 20 minutes

Doses for 4 people:

Ingredients:

Quinoa: 1 cup (200g)

Mixed vegetables (courgettes, cherry tomatoes,

peppers, carrots, etc.):

300g Cucumbers: 2 small

Fresh parsley leaves: 1 bunch

Lemon juice: 2 tablespoons

Extra virgin olive oil: 2 tablespoons

Salt and Pepper To Taste

Preparation:

Rinse the quinoa under running water and cook it following the instructions on the package. Let it cool. Cut the vegetables into cubes and the cucumbers into thin slices. In a large bowl, combine cooked quinoa, chopped vegetables, chopped parsley, lemon juice, olive oil, salt and pepper. Mix well. Let it rest in the refrigerator for at least 30 minutes before serving. Serve the salad cold or at room temperature. 7. Nutritional Values (per approximate serving): Calories: 250 kcal Protein: 8g Fat: 8g Carbohydrates: 35g Fibre: 6g Sugars: 4g Sodium: 300mg.

LIGHT MOZZARELLA IN CARROZZA WITH HOMEMADE MARINARA SAUCE

Preparation time: 15 minutes

Cooking times: 10 minutes

Doses for 4 people:

Ingredients:

Light mozzarella: 200g

Wholemeal sandwich bread: 8 slices

Eggs: 2, Skimmed milk: 100ml

Wholemeal flour: 50g

Peeled tomatoes: 400g

(for the marinara sauce)

Garlic: 2 cloves

Extra virgin olive oil: 2 tablespoons

Fresh basil: 1 bunch

Salt and Pepper To Taste

Preparation:

For the marinara sauce, heat the olive oil in a pan and sauté the chopped garlic. Add the peeled tomatoes and cook over medium heat for 10 minutes. Season with salt and pepper and add the chopped basil. Cut the mozzarella into slices and let them dry on absorbent paper. Prepare sandwiches with mozzarella inside. In a bowl, beat the eggs with the milk. Dip the bread slices in the flour, in the beaten egg and finally in the corn flour. Fry the bread slices in hot oil until golden brown. Serve the mozzarella in carrozza hot with the marinara sauce. 7. Nutrition Facts (per approximate serving, excluding marinara sauce): Calories: 280 kcal Protein: 14g Fat: 10g Carbohydrates: 35g Fiber: 5g Sugars: 4g Sodium: 400mg.

WHOLE CROUTTONS WITH RICOTTA AND HONEY

Preparation time: 10 minutes

Cooking times: 5 minutes

Doses for 4 people:

Ingredients:

Slices of wholemeal bread: 8 slices

Ricotta: 200g

Honey: 4 tablespoons

Chopped nuts (optional): 50g

Preparation:

Toast the slices of wholemeal bread until golden brown. Spread a generous amount of ricotta on each slice of toast. Add a drizzle of honey over the ricotta. Sprinkle with chopped walnuts if desired. Serve the crostini as an appetizer or snack. Nutritional values per approximate portion, considering 2 croutons): Calories: 150 kcal Proteins: 6g Fat: 5g Carbohydrates: 20g Fibre: 2g Sugars: 8g Sodium: 150mg

LEAN COOKED HAM AND FRESH FIGS

Preparation time: 10 minutes

Cooking times: 0 minutes

Doses for 4 people:

Ingredients:

Fresh figs: 8

Slices of lean cooked ham: 8 slices

Preparation:

Cut the figs into halves or quarters, depending on size. Wrap each slice of ham around the fig pieces. Arrange the morsels on a serving plate. Serve as an appetizer or snack. Nutritional values (per approximate portion, considering 2 slices of ham and 2 figs): Calories: 100 kcal Proteins: 6g Fat: 2g Carbohydrates: 15g Fibre: 2g Sugars: 12g Sodium: 300mg.

MARINATED OLIVES WITH AROMATIC HERBS AND LEMON

Preparation time: 10 minutes

Doses for 4 people:

Ingredients:

Black and green olives: 200g each

Grated lemon zest: from 1 lemon

Aromatic herbs (rosemary, thyme, oregano): 2 tablespoons

Ground black pepper: to taste

Extra virgin olive oil: 2 tablespoons

Preparation:

Rinse the olives well under running water. In a bowl, mix the olives with the grated lemon zest, herbs, black pepper and olive oil. Cover the bowl and leave to marinate in the refrigerator for at least 1 hour. Serve the marinated olives as an appetizer. 6. Nutritional Values (per approximate portion): Calories: 100 kcal Protein: 1g Fat: 10g Carbohydrates: 2g Fibre: 1g Sugars: 0g Sodium: 500mg

GRILLED AUBERGINES WITH DRIED TOMATOES AND FRESH BASIL

Preparation time: 15 minutes

Cooking times: 10 minutes

Doses for 4 people:

Ingredients:

Eggplant: 2 medium

Dried tomatoes in oil: 50g

Fresh basil: 20g

Extra virgin olive oil: 3 tablespoons

Salt and Pepper To Taste

Preparation:

Cut the aubergines into thin slices. Heat a grill and brush the eggplant slices with olive oil. Grill the aubergine slices until soft and streaked. Arrange the aubergine slices on a serving plate. Add the dried tomatoes and fresh basil leaves on top of the eggplant slices. Season with salt, pepper and a drizzle of olive oil. Serve the grilled eggplant as an appetizer or side dish. 7. Nutritional Values (per approximate serving): Calories: 120 kcal Protein: 2g Fat: 8g Carbohydrates: 10g Fibre: 4g Sugars: 3g Sodium: 200mg.

SMOKED SALMON CANAPÉS WITH SKYNNY CREAM CHEESE

Preparation time: 10 minutes

Doses for 4 people:

Ingredients:

Smoked salmon: 150g

Low-fat spreadable cheese: 150g

Sliced wholemeal bread: 8 slices

Chopped fresh chives:

2 tablespoons (optional)

Lemon: 1, thinly sliced

for garnish (optional)

Preparation:

Lightly toast the slices of wholemeal bread. Spread the low-fat cream cheese evenly on the toasted bread slices. Arrange the smoked salmon slices on top of the cheese. Garnish with chopped fresh chives and thin lemon slices, if desired. Serve as an appetizer or snack. 6. Nutritional Values (per approximate serving): Calories: 180 kcal Protein: 12g Fat: 8g Carbohydrates: 15g Fibre: 3g Sugars: 2g Sodium: 300mg.

CANNELLINI BEAN SALAD WITH NATURAL TUNA AND RED ONION

Preparation time: 15 minutes

Doses for 4 people:

Ingredients:

Canned cannellini beans, drained and rinsed: 400g

Natural tuna, drained: 200g

Red onion, sliced thinly: 1 medium

Chopped fresh parsley: 2 tablespoons

Lemon juice: 2 tablespoons

Extra virgin olive oil: 3 tablespoons

Salt and Pepper To Taste

Preparation:

In a large bowl, combine the cannellini beans, drained tuna, sliced red onion and chopped fresh parsley. Season with lemon juice, olive oil, salt and pepper. Stir gently to combine the ingredients. Let it rest in the refrigerator for at least 30 minutes before serving. Serve as a side dish or light main dish. 6. Nutritional Values (per approximate serving): Calories: 220 kcal Protein: 15g Fat: 8g Carbohydrates: 25g Fibre: 7g Sugars: 2g Sodium: 400mg.

CHICKEN BITES MARINATED WITH LEMON AND FRESH THYME

Preparation time: 15 minutes

(excluding marinades)

Cooking times: 15 minutes

Doses for 4 people:

Ingredients:

Chicken breast, cut into bite-sized pieces: 500g

Lemon juice: 4 tablespoons

Grated lemon zest: from 1 lemon

Fresh thyme, chopped: 2 tablespoons

Extra virgin olive oil: 2 tablespoons

Salt and Pepper To Taste

Preparation:

In a large bowl, combine the lemon juice, grated lemon zest, fresh thyme, olive oil, salt and pepper. Add the chicken tenders to the marinade and mix well to coat evenly. Leave to marinate in the refrigerator for at least 30 minutes. Heat a non-stick pan and cook the marinated chicken nuggets until golden and cooked through. Serve hot as a second course. 7. Nutritional Values (per approximate serving): Calories: 220 kcal Protein: 30g Fat: 10g Carbohydrates: 2g Fibre: 1g Sugars: 0g Sodium: 300mg.

GUACAMOLE WITH RAW VEGETABLES STICKS

Preparation time: 10 minutes

Doses for 4 people:

Ingredients:

Ripe avocado: 2

Tomatoes, small, diced: 2

Red onion, chopped

finely: 1 small

fresh coriander,

chopped: 2 tbsp

Lime juice: 1 lime

Salt and Pepper To Taste

Preparation:

In a bowl, mash the avocados until you get a creamy consistency. Add diced tomatoes, chopped red onion, chopped fresh cilantro and lime juice. Mix well and taste, adding salt and pepper to your taste. Serve with raw vegetable sticks such as carrots, celery, peppers, etc. 6. Nutritional Values (per approximate serving): Calories: 150 kcal Protein: 2g Fat: 12g Carbohydrates: 10g Fibre: 7g Sugars: 2g Sodium: 100mg.

POMEGRANATE SALAD, ARUGULA AND LIGHT PARMESAN FLAKES

Preparation time: 15 minutes

Doses for 4 people:

Ingredients:

Fresh Arugula: 150g

Pomegranate Seeds: 1 cup

Light parmesan, cut into flakes: 50g

Chopped nuts: 50g

Extra virgin olive oil: 2 tablespoons

Lemon juice: 1 tbsp

Salt and Pepper To Taste

Preparation:

In a large bowl, combine fresh arugula, pomegranate seeds, light parmesan flakes and chopped walnuts. Season with extra virgin olive oil, lemon juice, salt and pepper. Stir gently to combine the ingredients. Serve as an appetizer or side dish. 6. Nutritional Values (per approximate portion): Calories: 120 kcal Protein: 5g Fat: 8g Carbohydrates: 10g Fibre: 3g Sugars: 6g Sodium: 200mg.

WHOLEMEAL CROUTTONS WITH PORCINI MUSHROOMS AND FRESH PARSLEY

Preparation time: 20 minutes

Cooking times: 15 minutes

Doses for 4 people:

Ingredients:

Fresh porcini mushrooms,

cleaned and sliced: 300g

Sliced wholemeal bread: 8 slices

Garlic, minced: 2 cloves

Fresh parsley, chopped: 2 tablespoons

Extra virgin olive oil: 3 tablespoons

Salt and Pepper To Taste

Preparation:

Heat the olive oil in a pan and add the minced garlic. Add the sliced porcini mushrooms and cook until soft and golden. Season with salt and pepper. Toast the slices of wholemeal bread. Distribute the porcini mushrooms on the toasted croutons. Sprinkle with chopped fresh parsley. Serve as an appetizer or snack. 7. Nutritional Values (per approximate serving): Calories: 160 kcal Protein: 6g Fat: 7g Carbohydrates: 20g Fibre: 4g Sugars: 2g Sodium: 250mg.

CHICKEN MEATBALLS WITH HOMEMADE SWEET AND SOUR SAUCE

Preparation time: 20 minutes

Cooking times: 15 minutes

Doses for 4 people:

Ingredients:

Minced chicken breast: 500g

Wholemeal breadcrumbs: 50g

Egg: 1

Onion, finely chopped: 1 small

Garlic, minced: 2 cloves

Soy sauce: 2 tablespoons

Apple cider vinegar: 2 tablespoons

Grated fresh ginger: 1 teaspoon

Extra virgin olive oil: 2 tablespoons

Salt and Pepper To Taste

Preparation:

In a large bowl, mix the ground chicken breast with the breadcrumbs, egg, onion, garlic, salt and pepper. Form meatballs with your hands and set them aside. In a non-stick pan, heat the olive oil and cook the meatballs until golden and cooked through. Meanwhile, prepare the sweet and sour sauce by mixing the soy sauce, apple cider vinegar, and grated ginger in a small saucepan. Bring to the boil and reduce heat, simmering until sauce thickens slightly. Serve the meatballs with the sweet and sour sauce as a condiment. 7. Nutritional Values (per approximate serving): Calories: 250 kcal Protein: 25g Fat: 10g Carbohydrates: 15g Fibre: 2g Sugars: 6g Sodium: 400mg.

CHICKPEA SALAD WITH CHERRY TOMATOES AND CUCUMBERS

Preparation time: 15 minutes

Doses for 4 people:

Ingredients:

Canned cooked chickpeas, drained and rinsed: 400g

Cherry tomatoes, cut in half: 200g

Cucumbers, diced: 1 large

Red onion, thinly sliced:

1 small

Fresh parsley, chopped: 2 tablespoons

Lemon juice: 2 tablespoons

Extra virgin olive oil: 3 tablespoons

Salt and Pepper To Taste

Preparation:

In a large bowl, combine cooked chickpeas, cherry tomatoes, cucumbers, red onion and fresh parsley. Season with lemon juice, olive oil, salt and pepper. Stir gently to combine the ingredients. Let it rest in the refrigerator for at least 30 minutes before serving. Serve as a side dish or light main dish. 6. Nutritional Values (per approximate serving): Calories: 180 kcal Protein: 7g Fat: 8g Carbohydrates: 20g Fibre: 6g Sugars: 4g Sodium: 250mg.

TOMATOES STUFFED WITH TUNA AND CAPERS

Preparation time: 15 minutes

Doses for 4 people:

Ingredients:

Ripe, large tomatoes: 8

Tuna in oil,

drained: 200g

Capers, rinsed and

drained: 2 tablespoons

Fresh parsley,

chopped: 2 tbsp

Light mayonnaise: 4 tablespoons

Salt and Pepper To Taste

Preparation:

Cut off the top of the tomatoes and gently scoop out the pulp. In a bowl, mix the drained tuna, capers, chopped fresh parsley and mayonnaise. Stuff the tomatoes with the tuna mixture. Add salt and pepper if necessary. Serve as an appetizer or side dish. Nutritional Values (per serving): Calories: 120 kcal Proteins: 10g Fat: 5g Carbohydrates: 8g Fibre: 3g Sugars: 4g Sodium: 300mg.

WHOLE CROUTTONS WITH RICOTTA, LEAN RAW HAM AND ARUGULA

Preparation time: 10 minutes

Doses for 4 people:

Ingredients:

Sliced wholemeal bread: 8 slices

Fresh ricotta: 200g

Lean raw ham: 100g

Fresh Arugula: 50g

Extra virgin olive oil: 2 tablespoons

Salt and Pepper To Taste

Preparation:

Toast the slices of wholemeal bread. Spread the fresh ricotta on the toasted bread slices. Add a slice of lean raw ham to each slice of bread. Garnish with fresh arugula leaves. Season with a drizzle of extra virgin olive oil, salt and pepper to taste. Serve as an appetizer or snack. Nutritional values (per serving): Calories: 150 kcal Protein: 8g Fat: 6g Carbohydrates: 15g Fibre: 3g Sugars: 2g Sodium: 250mg.

SALMON TARTARE WITH AVOCADO AND MANGO

Preparation time: 20 minutes 3.

Doses for 4 people: 4.

Ingredients:

Fresh salmon, diced: 300g

Ripe avocado, diced: 1 large

Ripe mango, diced: 1 large

Red onion, finely chopped: 1 small

Lime juice: 2 tablespoons

Fresh coriander, chopped: 2 tablespoons

Fresh chili pepper, chopped

(optional): 1 small

Salt and Pepper To Taste

Preparation:

In a bowl, combine the diced salmon, diced avocado, diced mango and chopped red onion. Add lime juice, chopped fresh cilantro, and chopped fresh chili pepper, if desired. Stir gently to combine the ingredients. Add salt and pepper to your taste. Serve as a fresh starter or main course. Nutritional values (per serving): Calories: 250 kcal Protein: 20g Fat: 12g Carbohydrates: 15g Fibre: 5g Sugars: 8g Sodium: 150mg

BAKED POTATOES WITH ROSEMARY FRESH AND GARLIC

Preparation time: 10 minutes

Cooking times: 30/40 minutes

Doses for 4 people:

Ingredients:

Medium potatoes, washed and cut into segments: 800g

Garlic, crushed: 4 cloves

Rosemary sprigs fresh: 45 sprigs

Extra virgin olive oil: 3 tablespoons

Salt and Pepper To Taste

Preparation:

Preheat the oven to 200°C. In a large bowl, combine the potato wedges with the crushed garlic, fresh rosemary sprigs, olive oil, salt and pepper. Mix well to coat the potatoes evenly. Spread the potatoes on a baking sheet, making sure to spread them in an even layer. Bake in the preheated oven for 3040 minutes or until the potatoes are golden brown and tender inside. Serve hot as a side dish or main course. For nutritional values, you may want to calculate them based on serving sizes and the exact ingredients used. nutritional values (per serving): Calories: 180 kcal Proteins: 3g Fat: 7g Carbohydrates: 25g Fibre: 4g Sugars: 2g Sodium: 10mg.

WHOLE CROUTTONS WITH CONFIT TOMATOES AND BASIL PESTO

Preparation time: 15 minutes

Cooking times: 1 hour

Doses for 4 people:

Ingredients:

Cherry tomatoes: 500g

Garlic: 2 cloves

Extra virgin olive oil: 4 tablespoons

Brown sugar: 1 tbsp

Salt and Pepper To Taste

Sliced wholemeal bread: 8 slices

Basil pesto: 4 tablespoons

Preparation:

Cut the cherry tomatoes in half and place them on a baking tray lined with baking paper. Add whole garlic cloves and season with olive oil, sugar, salt and pepper. Cook in a preheated oven at 120°C for about 1 hour until the cherry tomatoes have wilted. Toast the slices of wholemeal bread. Spread the basil pesto on the bread slices and add the confit tomatoes. Serve as an appetizer or appetizer. Nutritional values (per serving): Calories: 180 kcal Protein: 4g Fat: 8g Carbohydrates: 22g Fibre: 3g Sugars: 4g Sodium: 250mg.

ORANGE BLACK OLIVES AND FENNEL SALAD,

Preparation time: 15 minutes

Doses for 4 people:

Ingredients:

Oranges: 4

Black olives: 100g

Fennel: 2

Extra virgin olive oil: 3 tablespoons

Lemon juice: 2 tablespoons

Fresh parsley,

chopped: 2 tbsp

Salt and Pepper To Taste

Preparation:

Peel the oranges and cut them into slices. Cut the fennel into thin slices. Arrange the orange and fennel slices on a serving plate. Add the black olives. Season with olive oil, lemon juice, fresh parsley, salt and pepper. Serve as an appetizer or side dish.

nutritional values (per serving): Calories: 120 kcal Proteins: 2g Fat: 7g Carbohydrates: 15g Fibre: 5g Sugars: 8g Sodium: 200mg.

WHOLE WHOLE CORN FRIES WITH LIGHT SPICY SAUCE

Preparation time: 20 minutes

Cooking times: 15 minutes

Doses for 4 people:

Ingredients:

Wholemeal corn flour: 1 cup

Eggs: 2

Skim milk: 1/2 cup

Canned sweet corn, drained: 1/2 cup

Green chilli, finely chopped: 1 chilli

Red onion, finely chopped: 1/4 cup

Fresh parsley, chopped: 2 tablespoons

Extra virgin olive oil: 2 tablespoons

Salt and Pepper To Taste

Light spicy sauce to accompany

Preparation:

In a large bowl, mix the whole-wheat cornmeal with the eggs and milk until smooth. Add the sweet corn, green chile, red onion and parsley. Mix well. Heat the olive oil in a nonstick skillet over medium heat. Pour a ladle of batter into the hot pan to form pancakes. Cook for 23 minutes per side or until golden and crispy. Drain the pancakes on absorbent paper to remove excess oil. Serve hot with a light spicy sauce. nutritional values (per serving): Calories: 180 kcal Proteins: 6g Fat: 8g Carbohydrates: 20g Fibre: 3g Sugars: 2g Sodium: 200mg

SMOKED SALMON ROLLS AND LIGHT SPREADABLE CHEESE ROLLS

Preparation time: 15 minutes

Doses for 4 people:

Ingredients:

Smoked salmon,

cut into thin slices: 200g

Light spreadable cheese: 100g

Fresh rocket: 1 bunch

Lemon juice: 2 tablespoons

Ground black pepper to taste

Chives, finely chopped:

1 tablespoon (optional)

Preparation:

Lay out the smoked salmon slices on a flat surface. Spread light cream cheese on each slice of salmon. Add a few arugula leaves to each slice. Gently roll the salmon to form rolls. Drizzle a little lemon juice over the rolls and sprinkle with ground black pepper and chives, if desired. Serve the salmon rolls as an appetizer or light snack. nutritional values (per serving): Calories: 150 kcal Proteins: 10g Fat: 7g Carbohydrates: 5g Fibre: 1g Sugars: 2g Sodium: 250mg.

WHOLE CROUTTONS WITH LIGHT CREAM CHEESE AND ROASTED PEPPERS

Preparation time: 15 minutes

Cooking times: 20 minutes

Doses for 4 people:

Ingredients:

Red and yellow peppers,

cut into strips: 2 pieces

Light spreadable cheese: 200g

Wholemeal croutons: 8 pieces

Extra virgin olive oil: 2 tablespoons

Salt and Pepper To Taste

Fresh basil to decorate

Preparation:

Preheat the oven to 200°C. Arrange the strips of peppers on a baking tray and sprinkle them with a drizzle of olive oil, salt and pepper. Bake the peppers in the oven for about 1520 minutes or until soft and lightly browned. Spread the cream cheese on the wholemeal croutons. Add the roasted pepper strips on top of the cream cheese. Decorate with fresh basil leaves. Serve as an appetizer or appetizer. Nutritional values (per serving): Calories: 150 kcal Protein: 5g Fat: 8g Carbohydrates: 15g Fiber: 2g Sugars: 3g Sodium: 200mg

CARPACCIO OF MIXED VEGETABLES WITH EXTRA VIRGIN OLIVE OIL AND LEMON

Preparation time: 15 minutes

Doses for 4 people:

Ingredients:

Zucchini, cut into thin slices: 2 pieces

Eggplant, cut into thin slices: 1 piece

Red and yellow peppers, cut into

thin slices: 1 piece each Mushrooms

champignons, cut into thin slices: 200g

Extra virgin olive oil: 3 tablespoons

Lemon juice: 2 tablespoons

Salt and Pepper To Taste

Grated Parmesan cheese

(optional) to serve

Preparation:

Arrange the vegetable slices decoratively on a serving platter. Drizzle extra virgin olive oil and lemon juice over the vegetables. Season with salt and pepper to taste. If desired, sprinkle with grated parmesan. Serve as a fresh and light appetizer. nutritional values (per serving): Calories: 100 kcal Proteins: 3g Fat: 7g Carbohydrates: 8g Fibre: 3g Sugars: 4g Sodium: 150mg.

SALAD OF TOMATOES LIGHT MOZZARELLA AND BASIL

Preparation time: 10 minutes

Doses for 4 people:

Ingredients:

Ripe tomatoes, cut into slices: 4

Light mozzarella, cut into slices: 200g

Fresh basil leaves: 1 bunch

Extra virgin olive oil: 2 tablespoons

Balsamic vinegar: 1 tbsp

Salt and Pepper To Taste

Preparation:

Arrange the tomato and mozzarella slices alternating them on a serving plate. Place the fresh basil leaves between the layers of tomato and mozzarella. Season with extra virgin olive oil, balsamic vinegar, salt and pepper. Serve as a fresh appetizer or light side dish. Nutritional values (per serving): Calories: 120 kcal Proteins: 8g Fat: 7g Carbohydrates: 5g Fibre: 2g Sugars: 3g Sodium: 250mg

WHOLE CROUTTONS WITH TUNA MOUSSE AND CAPERS

Preparation time: 15 minutes

Cooking times: 10 minutes

Doses for 4 people:

Ingredients:

Tuna in oil, drained: 200g

Light spreadable cheese: 100g

Capers, rinsed and

drained: 2 tablespoons

Lemon juice: 1 tbsp

Wholemeal croutons: 8 pieces

Fresh parsley, chopped:

1 tablespoon (optional)

Preparation:

In a blender, blend the tuna with the spreadable cheese and lemon juice until you obtain a creamy consistency. Add the capers and mix well. Spread the tuna mousse on the wholemeal croutons. If desired, sprinkle with chopped fresh parsley. Serve as an appetizer or appetizer. Nutritional values (per serving): Calories: 90 kcal Protein: 6g Fat: 4g Carbohydrates: 6g Fibre: 1g Sugars: 1g Sodium: 200mg.

DRIED TOMATOES STUFFED
OF RICOTTA LIGHT AND BASIL

Preparation time: 15 minutes

Cooking times: 0 minutes

Doses for 4 people:

Ingredients:

Dried tomatoes in oil: 8 pieces

Light ricotta: 200g

Basil leaves

fresh: 1 bunch

Ground black pepper to taste

Preparation:

Drain the dried tomatoes from the oil and dry them gently with absorbent paper. Fill them with light ricotta. Add a fresh basil leaf to each stuffed tomato. Sprinkle with a pinch of ground black pepper. Serve as an appetizer or as part of a buffet. Nutritional values (per serving): Calories: 70 kcal Protein: 4g Fat: 3g Carbohydrates: 6g Fibre: 2g Sugars: 2g Sodium: 100mg

BAKED AUBERGINE MEATBALLS WITH TOMATO SAUCE WITHOUT ADDED SUGAR

Preparation time: 20 minutes

Cooking times: 25 minutes

Doses for 4 people:

Ingredients:

Eggplant, diced: 2 medium

Whole grain breadcrumbs: 1/2 cup

Light grated cheese: 1/4 cup

Egg, lightly beaten: 1

Tomato sauce without

added sugars: 1 cup

Chopped fresh parsley: 2 tablespoons

Salt and black pepper to taste

Preparation:

Preheat the oven to 200°C. In a bowl, combine the diced aubergines, breadcrumbs, grated cheese, egg, chopped parsley, salt and pepper. Shape meatballs with your hands and place them on a baking tray lined with baking paper. Bake for about 25 minutes or until the meatballs are golden brown and cooked through. Heat the tomato sauce without added sugar and serve it alongside the meatballs. You can garnish with some fresh chopped parsley before serving. Nutritional values (per serving): Calories: 90 kcal Proteins: 5g Fat: 3g Carbohydrates: 12g Fibre: 3g Sugars: 5g Sodium: 150mg.

WHOLEWHEAT PIE WITH SPINACH AND LIGHT RICOTTA

Preparation time: 20 minutes

Cooking times: 40 minutes

Doses for 4 people:

Ingredients:

Wholemeal puff pastry: 1 roll

Fresh spinach, washed and chopped: 200g

Light ricotta: 200g

Eggs: 2

Light grated cheese: 50g

Nutmeg: 1 pinch

Salt and Pepper To Taste

Preparation:

Preheat the oven to 180°C. Line a pie pan with wholemeal puff pastry. In a pan, fry the spinach in a little oil until wilted. Drain any excess liquid. In a bowl, mix the ricotta with the eggs, grated cheese, nutmeg, salt and pepper. Add the spinach to the ricotta and egg mixture and mix well. Pour the mixture onto the puff pastry and level the surface. Bake in the oven for about 35/40 minutes or until the cake is golden and cooked in the center. Serve hot or at room temperature. Nutritional values (per portion): Calories: 250 kcal Protein: 10g Fat: 15g Carbohydrates: 20g Fibre: 2g Sugars: 2g Sodium: 300mg

BROWN RICE SALAD WITH NATURAL TUNA, OLIVES AND CORN

Preparation time: 15 minutes

Doses for 4 people:

Ingredients:

Cooked brown rice: 2 cups

Natural tuna, drained: 200g

Canned corn, drained: 1/2 cup

Black olives, pitted: 1/4 cup

Red peppers, diced: 1/2 bell pepper

Cucumbers, diced: 1 cucumber

Red onion, finely chopped: 1/4 cup

Fresh parsley, chopped: 2 tablespoons

Lemon juice: 2 tablespoons

Extra virgin olive oil: 3 tablespoons

Salt and Pepper To Taste

Preparation:

In a large bowl, combine cooked brown rice, tuna, corn, olives, peppers, cucumbers, red onion and fresh parsley. Season with lemon juice, olive oil, salt and pepper. Mix all the ingredients well until they are evenly distributed. Cover and let rest in the refrigerator for at least 30 minutes before serving. Mix again before serving and add salt and pepper if necessary. Nutritional values (per serving): Calories: 300 kcal Protein: 15g Fat: 8g Carbohydrates: 40g Fibre: 5g Sugars: 2g Sodium: 400mg.

RECIPES
FIRST DISHES

WHOLE WHOLE SPAGHETTI WITH DRIED TOMATO PESTO

Preparation time: 10 minutes

Cooking times: 10/12 minutes

Doses for 4 people:

Ingredients:

Wholemeal spaghetti: 400g

Dried tomatoes in oil: 100g

Fresh basil: 1 bunch

Walnuts: 50g

Grated parmesan: 50g

Extra virgin olive oil: 4 tablespoons

Garlic: 2 cloves

Salt and Pepper To Taste

Preparation:

Boil the wholemeal spaghetti in plenty of salted water following the instructions on the package until they are al dente. Meanwhile, blend the sun-dried tomatoes, basil, walnuts, parmesan, olive oil, and garlic until smooth. Drain the spaghetti and season them with the prepared pesto. Add salt and pepper if necessary. Serve hot, possibly garnished with fresh basil and chopped walnuts. Nutritional Values (per serving): Calories: 450 kcal Proteins: 15g Fat: 20g Carbohydrates: 55g Fibre: 8g Sugars: 5g Sodium: 450mg

WHOLE WHOLE RISOTTO WITH MIXED MUSHROOMS

Preparation time: 10 minutes

Cooking times: 25/30 minutes

Doses for 4 people:

Ingredients:

Brown rice: 300g

Mixed mushrooms (e.g. champignons, porcini mushrooms, shiitake): 300g

Onion: 1 large

Vegetable broth: 1 litre

Dry white wine: 1/2 glass

Butter: 2 tablespoons

Grated Parmesan: 50g

Chopped fresh parsley: 2 tablespoons

Extra virgin olive oil: 2 tablespoons

Salt and Pepper To Taste

Preparation:

Finely chop the onion and cut the mushrooms into slices. In a pan, heat the extra virgin olive oil and add the chopped onion. Fry until it becomes transparent. Add the mushrooms and cook until golden brown and the liquid has evaporated. Add the brown rice and toast it for a few minutes, stirring constantly. Deglaze with white wine and let the alcohol evaporate. Gradually add the hot vegetable broth, one ladle at a time, stirring occasionally and adding more broth as it is absorbed.

Continue until the rice is cooked al dente and has absorbed most of the broth (about 25/30 minutes). Turn off the heat and stir in the risotto with the butter and grated parmesan. Season with salt and pepper, if necessary, and add the chopped fresh parsley. Let it rest for a few minutes before serving. Nutritional Values (per serving): Calories: 380 kcal Proteins: 10g Fat: 8g Carbohydrates: 65g Fibre: 7g Sugars: 3g Sodium: 600mg.

LENTIL SOUP WITH SPINACH

Preparation time: 10 minutes

Cooking times: 40 minutes

Doses for 4 people:

Ingredients:

Dried lentils: 1 cup

Fresh spinach: 200g

Onion: 1 large

Carrots: 2 medium

Celery: 2 stalks

Vegetable broth: 1 litre

Peeled tomatoes: 400g

Extra virgin olive oil: 2 tablespoons

Salt and Pepper To Taste

Preparation:

Finely chop the onion, carrots and celery. In a large pot, heat the olive oil and add the chopped vegetables. Cook until tender. Add the lentils and crushed peeled tomatoes. Mix well. Pour in the vegetable broth and bring to the boil. Reduce the heat and simmer for about 30/35 minutes or until the lentils are soft. Add the spinach and let it sweat in the soup for 5 minutes. Add salt and pepper to taste. Serve the soup hot, possibly accompanied by wholemeal bread croutons. Values (per serving): Calories: 250 kcal Protein: 14g Fat: 5g Carbohydrates: 40g Fibre: 12g Sugars: 8g Sodium: 700mg

WHOLEWHEAT PENNE WITH FRESH TOMATO SAUCE

Preparation time: 15 minutes

Cooking times: 15 minutes

Doses for 4 people:

Ingredients:

Wholemeal penne: 400g

Ripe fresh tomatoes: 6 large

Garlic: 3 cloves

Fresh basil: 1 bunch

Extra virgin olive oil: 3 tablespoons

Salt and Pepper To Taste

Preparation:

Finely chop the garlic and cut the tomatoes into cubes. In a pan, heat the olive oil and add the minced garlic. Lightly sauté the garlic until golden. Add the diced tomatoes and cook over medium heat for about 12 minutes or until the tomatoes break down and become a sauce. In the meantime, cook the wholemeal penne in plenty of salted water following the instructions on the package. When the penne are al dente, drain them and add them to the fresh tomato sauce. Season with salt and pepper to taste and add the chopped fresh basil leaves. Mix well and serve hot. Nutritional Values (per serving): Calories: 320 kcal Proteins: 10g Fat: 5g Carbohydrates: 60g Fibre: 8g Sugars: 5g Sodium: 400mg.

SPELLED WITH VEGETABLE SAUCE

Preparation time: 10 minutes

Cooking times: 30/35 minutes

Doses for 4 people:

Ingredients:

Pearled spelled: 300g

Ripe tomatoes: 4 large

Carrots: 2 medium Celery: 2 stalks

Onion: 1 large

Zucchini: 2 medium

Red peppers: 1 large

Tomato puree: 200ml

Vegetable broth: 500ml

Extra virgin olive oil: 3 tablespoons

Salt and Pepper To Taste

Preparation:

Finely chop the onion, carrots, celery, courgettes and peppers. In a large pot, heat the olive oil and add the chopped vegetables. Cook until tender. Add the peeled tomatoes and the tomato puree. Mix well. Pour in the vegetable broth and bring to the boil. Reduce the heat and let simmer for about 2025 minutes. In the meantime, cook the pearled spelled in plenty of salted water following the instructions on the package. When the spelled is cooked, drain it and add it to the vegetable ragout. Mix well and leave to flavor for a few minutes. Add salt and pepper to taste. Serve the spelled with the hot vegetable ragout, possibly garnished with fresh basil. Nutritional Values (per serving): Calories: 350 kcal Proteins: 10g Fat: 6g Carbohydrates: 65g Fibre: 12g Sugars: 10g Sodium: 600mg

BARLEY WITH COURGETTES AND TOMATOES

Preparation time: 10 minutes

Cooking times: 20/25 minutes

Doses for 4 people:

Ingredients:

Barley: 300g

Courgettes: 3 medium

Cherry tomatoes: 250g

Onion: 1 large

Garlic: 2 cloves

Vegetable broth: 600ml

Extra virgin olive oil: 2 tablespoons

Fresh basil: 1 bunch

Salt and Pepper To Taste

Preparation:

Finely chop the onion and garlic. Cut the courgettes into cubes and the cherry tomatoes in half. In a saucepan, heat the olive oil and add the chopped onion and garlic. Fry until they become transparent. Add the courgettes and cherry tomatoes and cook for a few minutes until the vegetables are slightly wilted. Add the barley and toast it for a couple of minutes. Pour in the hot vegetable broth, cover the pan and leave to cook over medium-low heat for approximately 2025 minutes, or until the barley is cooked and has absorbed the liquid. Add salt and pepper to taste. Serve the barley with courgettes and cherry tomatoes hot, garnished with fresh basil leaves. Nutritional Values (per serving): Calories: 320 kcal Proteins: 8g Fat: 5g Carbohydrates: 60g Fibre: 8g Sugars: 5g Sodium: 500mg.

WILD RICE WITH STEAMED BROCCOLI

Preparation time: 10 minutes

Cooking times: 35/40 minutes

Doses for 4 people:

Ingredients:

Wild rice: 300g

Broccoli: 1 bunch

Garlic: 2 cloves

Extra virgin olive oil:

3 tbsp

Salt and Pepper To Taste

Preparation:

Rinse the wild rice under running water. Place the wild rice in a pot and cover it with double the amount of cold water. Bring to the boil, then reduce the heat, cover and cook for about 35/40 minutes or until the rice is tender and has absorbed the water. In the meantime, cut the broccoli into florets and steam them for about 5/7 minutes until they become tender but still crunchy. In a pan, heat the olive oil and add the minced garlic. Saute the garlic until golden. Once cooked, combine the broccoli with the cooked wild rice and mix gently. Add salt and pepper to taste. Serve wild rice with hot steamed broccoli. Nutritional Values (per serving): Calories: 280 kcal Proteins: 8g Fat: 7g Carbohydrates: 50g Fibre: 6g Sugars: 3g Sodium: 300mg

BUCKWHEAT LINGUINE WITH ARUGULA PESTO

Preparation time: 15 minutes

Cooking times: 10 minutes

Doses for 4 people:

Ingredients:

Buckwheat linguine: 400g

Arugula: 100g

Almonds: 50g

Grated parmesan: 50g

Garlic: 2 cloves

Lemon juice: 1 tbsp

Extra virgin olive oil: 4 tablespoons

Salt and Pepper To Taste

Preparation:

Cook the buckwheat linguine in plenty of salted water following the instructions on the package. Drain them al dente. Meanwhile, prepare the rocket pesto. In a blender, combine the arugula, almonds, parmesan, garlic, lemon juice, and olive oil. Blend until you obtain a creamy consistency. If necessary, add a little water to achieve the desired consistency. Season the cooked linguine with the Arugula pesto and mix well. Add salt and pepper to taste. Serve the buckwheat linguine with Arugula pesto hot. Nutritional Values (per serving): Calories: 350 kcal Proteins: 10g Fat: 15g Carbohydrates: 45g Fibre: 7g Sugars: 3g Sodium: 350mg.

AUBERGINES AND SPINACH LASAGNA

Preparation time: 30 minutes

Cooking times: 45 minutes

Doses for 4 people:

Ingredients:

Aubergines: 2 large

Fresh spinach: 300g

Egg lasagne: 250g

Peeled tomatoes: 400g

Onion: 1 large

Garlic: 2 cloves

Ricotta cheese: 250g

Grated parmesan cheese: 100g

Mozzarella: 200g Olive oil

extra virgin: 3 tablespoons

Salt and Pepper To Taste

Preparation:

Cut the aubergines into thin slices and grill them on both sides until tender. Chop the onion and garlic and cook them in a pan with olive oil. Add the peeled tomatoes and cook for about 15 minutes. In a separate pan, cook the spinach until wilted. In a baking dish, alternate layers of grilled eggplant, lasagna, tomato sauce, spinach and ricotta cheese. Finish with a final layer of lasagna, tomato sauce and parmesan cheese. Bake in a preheated oven at 180°C for about 30 minutes, until the cheese is golden and the lasagna is hot and bubbly. Let it rest for a few minutes before serving. Nutritional Values (per serving): Calories: 380 kcal Proteins: 20g Fat: 15g Carbohydrates: 40g Fibre: 8g Sugars: 10g Sodium: 700mg.

KONJAC TAGLIATELLE WITH TOMATO AND BASIL SAUCE

Preparation time: 10 minutes

Cooking times: 15 minutes

Doses for 4 people:

Ingredients:

Konjac noodles: 400g

Peeled tomatoes: 400g

Garlic: 2 cloves

Fresh basil: 1 bunch

Extra virgin olive oil: 2 tablespoons

Salt and Pepper To Taste

Preparation:

Rinse the konjac tagliatelle well under running water and cook them in boiling water for 23 minutes. In a pan, heat the olive oil and fry the finely chopped garlic. Add the peeled tomatoes and cook for about 10 minutes, mashing them with a fork. Add the chopped fresh basil, salt and pepper. Add the drained konjac tagliatelle and sauté for a couple of minutes to absorb the seasoning. Serve hot, garnished with fresh basil leaves. Nutritional Values (per serving): Calories: 120 kcal Proteins: 2g Fat: 4g Carbohydrates: 20g Fibre: 10g Sugars: 5g Sodium: 500mg.

QUINOA WITH GRILLED VEGETABLES

Preparation time: 15 minutes

Cooking times: 20 minutes

Doses for 4 people:

Ingredients:

Quinoa: 1 cup approximately 200 g.

Eggplant: 1 large

Zucchini: 2 medium

Red peppers: 1 large

Red onion: 1 large

Cherry tomatoes: 200g

Extra virgin olive oil: 3 tablespoons

Lemon juice: 2 tablespoons

Salt and Pepper To Taste

Preparation:

Rinse the quinoa well under cold water. Cook the quinoa in lightly salted boiling water following the instructions on the package, about 15/20 minutes. Meanwhile, cut the aubergines, courgettes, peppers and onion into slices. Heat a grill or nonstick skillet and grill the vegetables until tender and lightly browned. In a large bowl, mix the cooked quinoa with the grilled vegetables. Add the cherry tomatoes cut in half. Season with olive oil, lemon juice, salt and pepper. Serve hot or cold as a main course or side dish. Nutritional Values (per serving): Calories: 250 kcal Proteins: 8g Fat: 8g Carbohydrates: 40g Fibre: 7g Sugars: 5g Sodium: 300mg.

WHOLE WHOLE RAVIOLI WITH RICOTTA AND SPINACH FILLING

Preparation time: 30 minutes

Cooking times: 10 minutes

Doses for 4 people:

Ingredients:

Wholemeal ravioli: 400g

Fresh ricotta: 250g

Fresh spinach: 200g

Grated parmesan: 50g

Nutmeg: to taste

Salt and Pepper To Taste

Preparation:

Boil the spinach in boiling salted water for 23 minutes. Drain and squeeze them well to remove excess water. In a large bowl, combine the boiled spinach, fresh ricotta, grated Parmesan, nutmeg, salt and pepper. Mix well until you obtain a homogeneous mixture. Roll out the ravioli dough and distribute the filling in small, evenly spaced quantities. Close the ravioli with another sheet of pasta, pressing the edges well to seal them. Cook the ravioli in plenty of boiling salted water for about 4/5 minutes, or until they float to the surface. Drain them with a slotted spoon and season them with your favorite sauce or a drizzle of olive oil. Nutritional Values (per serving): Calories: 350 kcal Proteins: 15g Fat: 10g Carbohydrates: 50g Fibre: 8g Sugars: 3g Sodium: 400mg.

PUMPKIN SPAGHETTI WITH TOMATO SAUCE

Preparation time: 15 minutes

Cooking times: 20 minutes

Doses for 4 people:

Ingredients:

Pumpkin: 1 large

Ripe tomatoes: 4 large

Garlic: 3 cloves

Fresh basil: 1 bunch

Extra virgin olive oil: 3 tablespoons

Salt and Pepper To Taste

Preparation:

Cut the pumpkin in half and remove the seeds. Using a peeler or a potato peeler, make spaghetti from the pumpkin pulp. In a pan, heat the olive oil and add the minced garlic. Lightly brown the garlic. Add the diced tomatoes and cook for about 10/15 minutes until they become soft and a sauce forms. Add the chopped fresh basil and season with salt and pepper. In a separate pan, cook the spaghetti squash in lightly salted water for about 5/7 minutes, until al dente. Drain the spaghetti squash and season them with the tomato sauce. Serve hot, garnished with fresh basil. Nutritional Values (per serving): Calories: 150 kcal Proteins: 3g Fat: 7g Carbohydrates: 20g Fibre: 5g Sugars: 8g Sodium: 300mg

SWEET POTATO GNOCCHI WITH BASIL PESTO

Preparation time: 30 minutes

Cooking times: 10 minutes

Doses for 4 people:

Ingredients:

Sweet potatoes: 4 medium

Whole wheat flour: 1 cup

Eggs: 1 large

Fresh basil: 1 bunch

Walnuts: 50g

Grated parmesan: 50g

Extra virgin olive oil: 3 tablespoons

Garlic: 2 cloves

Salt and Pepper To Taste

Preparation:

Cook sweet potatoes in their skins in boiling water until tender. Drain and let them cool slightly. Remove the skin from the sweet potatoes and mash them with a potato masher or fork in a large bowl. Add the wholemeal flour, egg, salt and pepper to the mashed potatoes and mix until smooth. Divide the dough into small portions and shape into gnocchi. In a saucepan, bring lightly salted water to a boil. Cook the gnocchi in boiling water until they float to the surface. Meanwhile, make the basil pesto by blending fresh basil, walnuts, parmesan, garlic, olive oil, salt, and pepper in a blender. Drain the gnocchi and season them with the basil pesto. Serve hot, garnished with chopped walnuts and grated parmesan. Nutritional Values (per serving): Calories: 320 kcal Proteins: 8g Fat: 12g Carbohydrates: 45g Fibre: 6g Sugars: 8g Sodium: 400mg.

SPELLED RISOTTO WITH SAFFRON AND ASPARAGUS

Preparation time: 10 minutes

Cooking times: 30 minutes

Doses for 4 people:

Ingredients:

Spelled: 300g

Asparagus: 1 bunch

Saffron: 1 sachet

Vegetable broth: 1 litre

Onion: 1 large

Dry white wine: 1/2 glass

Extra virgin olive oil: 2 tablespoons

Salt and Pepper To Taste

Preparation:

Cut the asparagus into pieces and steam them until tender but crunchy. In a pan, heat the olive oil and fry the finely chopped onion. Add the spelled and toast it lightly for a few minutes. Blend with the dry white wine and add the saffron. Gradually add the hot vegetable broth, stirring occasionally, until the spelled is cooked and the risotto has reached a creamy consistency. Add the cooked asparagus to the risotto, season with salt and pepper. Serve hot, garnished with a pinch of saffron on top of each dish. Nutritional Values (per serving): Calories: 300 kcal Proteins: 10g Fat: 5g Carbohydrates: 55g Fibre: 8g Sugars: 3g Sodium: 600mg

COURGETTE SPAGHETTI OMELETTE WITH TOMATOES

Preparation time: 15 minutes

Cooking times: 15 minutes

Doses for 4 people:

Ingredients:

Courgettes: 4 medium

Eggs: 6 large

Cherry tomatoes: 200g

Grated parmesan: 50g

Onion: 1 medium

Extra virgin olive oil: 2 tablespoons

Fresh parsley: to taste

Salt and Pepper To Taste

Preparation:

Cut the courgettes into spaghetti using a spiralizer. In a non-stick pan, heat the olive oil and add the finely chopped onion. Sauté the onion. Add the courgette spaghetti and the cherry tomatoes cut in half. Cook for about 5/7 minutes until the courgettes are tender. In a bowl, beat the eggs with the grated parmesan, chopped fresh parsley, salt and pepper. Pour the beaten eggs over the zucchini and cherry tomato spaghetti in the pan. Cook over medium-low heat until the omelette is set on the edges but still slightly liquid in the center. Transfer the pan under the oven grill for 3/5 minutes or until the surface is golden and the omelette is completely cooked. Cut the omelette into wedges and serve hot or at room temperature. Nutritional Values (per serving): Calories: 180 kcal Proteins: 12g Fat: 10g Carbohydrates: 12g Fibre: 3g Sugars: 4g Sodium: 300mg.

BASMATI RICE WITH VEGETABLE CURRY

Preparation time: 15 minutes

Cooking times: 20 minutes

Doses for 4 people:

Ingredients:

Basmati rice: 2 cups 400 gr.

Mixed vegetables (e.g. carrots, peas, peppers, onion): 500g

Coconut milk: 1 can

Curry powder: 2 tbsp

Garlic: 2 cloves

Grated fresh ginger: 1 tbsp

Extra virgin olive oil: 2 tablespoons

Salt and Pepper To Taste

Preparation:

Cook the basmati rice according to the package instructions. In a large skillet, heat the olive oil and add the minced garlic and grated ginger. Fry for a minute. Add the chopped vegetables and cook until tender but crisp. Pour the coconut milk into the pan with the vegetables, add the curry powder, salt and pepper. Mix well and leave to cook over medium heat for about 5/7 minutes. Add the basmati rice to the pan with the vegetable curry and stir gently until the rice is well seasoned with the curry. Serve hot and garnish with fresh herbs if desired. Nutritional Values (per serving): Calories: 300 kcal Proteins: 7g Fat: 10g Carbohydrates: 45g Fibre: 6g Sugars: 5g Sodium: 400mg

WHOLE WHOLE COUSCOUS WITH CHICKPEAS AND TOMATO

Preparation time: 10 minutes

Cooking times: 10 minutes

Doses for 4 people:

Ingredients:

Wholemeal couscous: 2 cups approximately 200 gr.

Cooked chickpeas: 1 can

Cherry tomatoes: 250g

Red onion: 1 medium

Fresh parsley: to taste

Extra virgin olive oil: 2 tablespoons

Lemon juice: 2 tablespoons

Salt and Pepper To Taste

Preparation:

Prepare wholemeal couscous following the instructions on the package. In a pan, heat the olive oil and add the finely chopped red onion. Sauté for a few minutes until translucent. Add the cherry tomatoes cut in half and the cooked chickpeas. Cook for another 5/7 minutes until the cherry tomatoes begin to release their juices. In a large bowl, combine the prepared wholemeal couscous with the cherry tomatoes, chickpeas and onion. Season with lemon juice, salt, pepper and chopped fresh parsley. Serve hot or at room temperature as a side dish or main course. Nutritional Values (per serving): Calories: 250 kcal Proteins: 8g Fat: 5g Carbohydrates: 40g Fibre: 8g Sugars: 5g Sodium: 300mg.

OAT FETTUCCINE WITH MUSHROOM CREAM

Preparation time: 15 minutes

Cooking times: 20 minutes

Doses for 4 people:

Ingredients:

Oat fettuccine: 400g

Mixed mushrooms (e.g. champignons, porcini mushrooms): 500g

Onion: 1 medium

Garlic: 2 cloves

Vegetable broth: 500ml

Vegetable cream: 200ml

Extra virgin olive oil: 2 tablespoons

Fresh parsley: to taste

Salt and Pepper To Taste

Preparation:

Cook the oat fettuccine in plenty of salted water following the instructions on the package. Drain them al dente and reserve a little of the cooking water. In a pan, heat the olive oil and add the chopped onion and minced garlic. Fry until golden brown. Add the sliced mushrooms and cook until golden brown and have released their juices. Add the vegetable broth and cook for 10 minutes. Blend the mushrooms with an immersion blender until you obtain a smooth cream. Add the vegetable cream to the mushroom cream and mix well. Combine the oat fettuccine with the mushroom cream, adding a little cooking water if necessary to obtain a creamy consistency. Season with salt and pepper, and serve hot, garnished with fresh chopped parsley. Nutritional Values (per serving): Calories: 350 kcal Proteins: 10g Fat: 12g Carbohydrates: 50g Fibre: 8g Sugars: 5g Sodium: 400mg.

RICE VERMICELLI WITH PRAWNS AND VEGETABLES

Preparation time: 20 minutes

Cooking times: 15 minutes

Doses for 4 people:

Ingredients:

Rice vermicelli: 300g

Peeled and cleaned prawns: 300g

Mixed vegetables julienned (e.g. carrots, courgettes, peppers): 500g

Soy sauce: 3 tablespoons

Garlic: 2 cloves

Grated fresh ginger: 1 tbsp

Sesame oil: 2 tablespoons

Fresh chili pepper (optional): to taste

Fresh parsley: to taste

Salt and Pepper To Taste

Preparation:

Cook the rice vermicelli in boiling salted water following the instructions on the package. Drain and rinse with cold water to stop cooking. In a pan, heat the sesame oil and add the minced garlic, grated ginger and fresh chili pepper (if using). Fry for a minute. Add the shrimp and cook until pink and cooked through. Add julienned vegetables and cook until tender but crisp. Add the rice vermicelli to the pan with the shrimp and vegetables. Add the soy sauce, season with salt and pepper, and mix well to evenly distribute the flavors. Serve hot, garnished with fresh chopped parsley. Nutritional Values (per serving): Calories: 320 kcal Proteins: 20g Fat: 8g Carbohydrates: 45g Fibre: 6g Sugars: 3g Sodium: 600mg.

POLENTA WITH TOMATO SAUCE AND MUSHROOMS

Preparation time: 10 minutes

Cooking times: 30 minutes

Doses for 4 people:

Ingredients:

Instant polenta: 250g

Mixed mushrooms (e.g. champignons, porcini mushrooms): 400g

Peeled tomatoes: 400g

Onion: 1 medium

Garlic: 2 cloves

Vegetable broth: 500ml

Extra virgin olive oil: 2 tablespoons

Fresh parsley: to taste

Salt and Pepper To Taste

Preparation:

Prepare instant polenta according to package instructions. Pour the cooked polenta into a pan and leave to cool. In a pan, heat the olive oil and add the chopped onion and minced garlic. Fry until golden brown. Add the sliced mushrooms and cook until golden. Add the peeled tomatoes and mash them with a fork. Cook for about 15/20 minutes until the ragù thickens slightly. Season with salt and pepper, and add chopped fresh parsley. Cut the polenta into pieces and serve hot with the tomato and mushroom ragù on top. Nutritional Values (per serving): Calories: 350 kcal Proteins: 8g Fat: 10g Carbohydrates: 55g Fibre: 10g Sugars: 5g Sodium: 600mg

LENTIL PASTA WITH TOMATOES AND BASIL

Preparation time: 15 minutes

Cooking times: 10 minutes

Doses for 4 people:

Ingredients:

Lentil pasta: 300g

Cherry tomatoes: 300g

Garlic: 2 cloves

Fresh basil: to taste

Extra virgin olive oil: 2 tablespoons

Salt and Pepper To Taste

Preparation:

Cook the lentil pasta in plenty of salted water following the instructions on the package. Drain and reserve some of the cooking water. In a pan, heat the olive oil and add the minced garlic. Fry until golden. Add the halved cherry tomatoes and cook for a few minutes until they start to release their juices. Add the lentil paste to the pan with the cherry tomatoes and mix well. If necessary, add a little pasta cooking water to create a creamy consistency. Season with salt and pepper, and garnish with fresh basil leaves. Serve hot and tasty! Nutritional Values (per serving): Calories: 320 kcal Proteins: 15g Fat: 8g Carbohydrates: 50g Fibre: 10g Sugars: 5g Sodium: 400mg.

SQUID INK RISOTTO WITH PRAWNS

Preparation time: 15 minutes

Cooking times: 20 minutes

Doses for 4 people:

Ingredients:

Rice for risotto: 320g

Squid ink (bags): 2

Shelled shrimp: 300g

Vegetable broth: 1 litre

Onion: 1 medium

Dry white wine: 120ml

Butter: 50g

Grated parmesan: 50g

Extra virgin olive oil: 2 tablespoons

Salt and Pepper To Taste

Preparation:

In a saucepan, heat the vegetable broth and keep it warm. In a pan, fry the finely chopped onion in the olive oil. Add the rice and toast it for a few minutes. Deglaze with white wine and let the alcohol evaporate. Add the previously cleaned and chopped cuttlefish ink. Add a ladle of hot broth at a time, stirring occasionally, until the rice is cooked al dente. Halfway through cooking, add the peeled shrimp. Stir the risotto with the butter and grated parmesan. Add salt and pepper, if necessary, and serve hot. Nutritional Values (per serving): Calories: 400 kcal Proteins: 18g Fat: 12g Carbohydrates: 55g Fibre: 2g Sugars: 1g Sodium: 700mg

KAMUT CAPELLINI WITH GARLIC, OIL AND CHILI PEPPER

Preparation time: 5 minutes

Cooking times: 8 minutes

Doses for 4 people:

Ingredients:

Kamut Capellini: 340 g

Garlic: 4 cloves

Fresh chili pepper: 1 piece

Extra virgin olive oil: 4 tablespoons

Fresh parsley: to taste

Salt to taste

Preparation:

Cook the kamut Capellini in plenty of salted water following the instructions on the package. Meanwhile, in a pan, heat the olive oil and add the chopped garlic and the fresh chili pepper cut into thin slices. Saute the garlic and chilli over medium heat until the garlic is golden brown. Drain the Capellini al dente and transfer them to the pan with the oil, garlic and chilli. Sauté the Capellini for a minute to add flavour. Add the chopped fresh parsley and season with salt, if necessary. Serve hot and tasty! Nutritional Values (per serving): Calories: 350 kcal Proteins: 10g Fat: 12g Carbohydrates: 50g Fibre: 8g Sugars: 2g Sodium: 400mg.

WHOLE BUTTERFLIES WITH SPINACH AND WALNUT PESTO

Preparation time: 15 minutes

Cooking times: 10 minutes

Doses for 4 people:

Ingredients:

Wholemeal farfalle: 350g

Fresh spinach: 200g

Walnuts: 50g

Garlic: 2 cloves

Extra virgin olive oil: 4 tablespoons

Grated parmesan: 50g

Salt and Pepper To Taste

Preparation:

Cook the whole farfalle in plenty of salted water following the instructions on the package. Drain them al dente and reserve a little of the cooking water. In a pan, heat the olive oil and add the fresh spinach. Cook them until they wilt. Add the spinach and walnuts to a blender, along with the minced garlic and grated parmesan. Blend everything until you obtain a homogeneous consistency. Dilute the pesto with a little of the farfalle cooking water, if necessary. Combine the farfalle with the spinach and walnut pesto, mixing well to evenly distribute the sauce. Season with salt and pepper, and serve hot. Nutritional Values (per serving): Calories: 380 kcal Proteins: 12g Fat: 15g Carbohydrates: 50g Fibre: 8g Sugars: 2g Sodium: 500mg

QUINOA AND BEAN MINESTRONE

Preparation time: 15 minutes

Cooking times: 30 minutes

Doses for 4 people:

Ingredients:

Quinoa: 150g

Mixed beans (cannellini, borlotti, etc.): 400g

Carrots: 2 medium

Celery: 2 stalks

Onion: 1 medium

Ripe tomatoes: 2 large

Vegetable broth: 1 litre

Extra virgin olive oil: 2 tablespoons

Fresh parsley: to taste

Salt and Pepper To Taste

Preparation:

In a saucepan, heat the olive oil and add the chopped onion, diced carrots and chopped celery. Sauté until the vegetables are wilted. Add the diced ripe tomatoes and cook for a few minutes. Pour the vegetable broth into the pot and bring to the boil. Add the quinoa and drained and rinsed beans. Cook over medium-low heat until the quinoa is cooked and the beans are tender. Season with salt and pepper, if necessary, and garnish with chopped fresh parsley. Serve hot and enjoy this flavorful and nutritious soup! Nutritional Values (per serving): Calories: 320 kcal Proteins: 12g Fat: 8g Carbohydrates: 50g Fibre: 10g Sugars: 5g Sodium: 600mg.

BUCKWHEAT SPAGHETTI WITH VEGETABLE SAUCE

Preparation time: 15 minutes

Cooking times: 20 minutes

Doses for 4 people:

Ingredients:

Buckwheat spaghetti: 340g

Mixed vegetables of your choice (courgettes, aubergines, peppers, carrots): 500g

Peeled tomatoes: 400g

Onion: 1 medium

Garlic: 2 cloves

Fresh parsley: to taste

Extra virgin olive oil: 2 tablespoons

Salt and Pepper To Taste

Preparation:

Cut the vegetables into cubes or julienne strips. In a pan, heat the olive oil and add the chopped onion and minced garlic. Fry until golden brown. Add the chopped vegetables and cook until soft. Add the peeled tomatoes and mash them with a fork. Cook for about 15/20 minutes until the ragù thickens slightly. Season with salt and pepper, and add chopped fresh parsley. In the meantime, cook the buckwheat spaghetti in plenty of salted water following the instructions on the package. Drain the spaghetti al dente and season them with the vegetable ragù. Serve hot, garnished with a little chopped fresh parsley. Nutritional Values (per serving): Calories: 350 kcal Proteins: 10g Fat: 8g Carbohydrates: 60g Fibre: 12g Sugars: 8g Sodium: 500mg

PUMPKIN RAVIOLI WITH BUTTER AND SAGE

Preparation time: 30 minutes

Cooking times: 5 minutes

Doses for 4 people:

Ingredients:

Pumpkin ravioli: 400g

Pumpkin: 500g

Butter: 50g

Fresh sage leaves: 10/12

Grated parmesan: to taste

Salt to taste

Preparation:

Boil the pumpkin until soft, then mash it with a fork or blend it until it becomes a puree. Cook the pumpkin ravioli in plenty of salted water following the instructions on the package. Drain them al dente. In a skillet, melt the butter over medium heat until it starts to turn golden. Add the sage leaves and let them brown slightly. Add the drained pumpkin ravioli to the skillet with the butter and sage, stirring gently to distribute the seasoning. Serve the ravioli hot, sprinkling them with grated parmesan to taste. Nutritional Values (per serving): Calories: 400 kcal Proteins: 12g Fat: 15g Carbohydrates: 55g Fibre: 8g Sugars: 5g Sodium: 400mg.

BARLEY AND VEGETABLE SOUP

Preparation time: 15 minutes

Cooking times: 30 minutes

Doses for 4 people:

Ingredients:

Barley: 150g

Mixed vegetables of your choice (carrots, celery, potatoes, courgettes): 500g

Onion: 1 medium

Garlic: 2 cloves

Vegetable broth: 1 litre

Fresh parsley: to taste

Extra virgin olive oil: 2 tablespoons

Salt and Pepper To Taste

Preparation:

Cut the vegetables into cubes or small pieces. In a saucepan, heat the olive oil and add the chopped onion and minced garlic. Fry until golden brown. Add the chopped vegetables and cook until soft. Add the barley and vegetable broth. Bring to the boil and then reduce the heat. Let simmer until the orzo is cooked and the vegetables are tender. Season with salt and pepper, and add chopped fresh parsley. Serve hot, accompanied by a slice of wholemeal bread, if you prefer. Nutritional Values (per serving): Calories: 300 kcal Proteins: 8g Fat: 6g Carbohydrates: 50g Fibre: 10g Sugars: 5g Sodium: 600mg

CHICKPEA LINGUINE WITH TOMATOES AND BLACK OLIVES

Preparation time: 10 minutes

Cooking times: 15 minutes

Doses for 4 people:

Ingredients:

Chickpea linguine: 320g

Cherry tomatoes: 250g

Black olives: 100g

Garlic: 2 cloves

Extra virgin olive oil: 3 tablespoons

Chili pepper (optional): to taste

Fresh basil: to taste

Salt to taste

Preparation:

Cook the chickpea linguine in plenty of salted water following the instructions on the package. Drain them al dente. In a pan, heat the olive oil and add the minced garlic and, if desired, the chili pepper. Add the cherry tomatoes cut in half and the pitted black olives. Cook for a few minutes until the cherry tomatoes begin to release their juices. Add the drained chickpea linguine directly to the pan with the seasoning. Add salt if necessary. Serve the linguine hot, garnished with fresh basil to taste. Nutritional Values (per serving): Calories: 380 kcal Proteins: 14g Fat: 10g Carbohydrates: 60g Fibre: 12g Sugars: 5g Sodium: 400mg.

RECIPES
SECOND DISHES

LEMON CHICKEN BREAST WITH BROCCOLETTI

Preparation time: 10 minutes

Cooking times: 20 minutes

Doses for 4 people:

Ingredients:

Chicken breast: 4 fillets (about 600g)

Lemon: 2 large (juice

and grated zest)

Garlic: 3 cloves, finely chopped

Broccoli: 500g, cleaned and cut into pieces

Extra virgin olive oil: 3 tablespoons

Fresh parsley: to taste

Salt and Pepper To Taste

Preparation:

Preheat the oven to 200°C. In a bowl, mix the lemon juice and grated zest with the minced garlic, salt, pepper and olive oil. Place the chicken breast fillets on a baking tray and brush them with the lemon marinade. Bake the chicken for about 20 minutes or until cooked through and golden brown. Meanwhile, cook the broccoli in boiling salted water for about 7 minutes or until tender but crisp. Drain the broccoli and season it with a drizzle of olive oil and salt. Serve the lemon chicken breast with the hot broccoli, garnished with chopped fresh parsley. Nutritional Values (per serving): Calories: 300 kcal Proteins: 40g Fat: 12g Carbohydrates: 10g Fibre: 5g Sugars: 2g Sodium: 500mg

GRILLED SALMON WITH AVOCADO SAUCE

Preparation time: 15 minutes

Cooking times: 10 minutes

Doses for 4 people:

Ingredients:

Salmon fillets: 4 (about 800g)

Ripe avocado: 2 large

Lemon juice: 2 tablespoons

Garlic: 1 clove, finely chopped

Fresh chili pepper: 1 piece, finely chopped (optional)

Salt and Pepper To Taste

Extra virgin olive oil: 2 tablespoons

Preparation:

Preheat the grill. In a bowl, mash the avocados and mix with the lemon juice, minced garlic, chili pepper (if desired), salt and pepper. Brush the salmon fillets lightly with olive oil and season with salt and pepper. Grill the salmon for about 4 to 5 minutes per side or until cooked but still juicy. Serve the salmon hot, accompanied by the avocado sauce. Nutritional Values (per serving): Calories: 350 kcal Protein: 30g Fat: 20g Carbohydrates: 10g Fibre: 8g Sugars: 2g Sodium: 500mg.

VEAL PIZZAIOLA WITH TOMATOES AND OREGANO

Preparation time: 15 minutes

Cooking times: 30 minutes

Doses for 4 people:

Ingredients:

Veal slices: 600g

Peeled tomatoes: 400g

Garlic: 3 cloves, finely chopped

Fresh or dried oregano: 2 tablespoons

Extra virgin olive oil: 3 tablespoons

Salt and Pepper To Taste

Preparation:

Heat the olive oil in a non-stick pan and brown the veal slices on both sides until they are golden brown. Remove the veal from the pan and set aside. In the same pan, add the minced garlic and fry until golden. Add the peeled tomatoes, oregano, salt and pepper. Lightly mash the tomatoes with a fork. Cook over medium-low heat for about 15 minutes or until the sauce thickens. Add the veal slices to the sauce, cover the pan and cook for a further 10 to 15 minutes or until the meat is tender. Serve the veal pizzaiola hot, garnished with a little fresh oregano. Nutritional Values (per serving): Calories: 350 kcal Proteins: 40g Fat: 15g Carbohydrates: 10g Fibre: 3g Sugars: 5g Sodium: 600mg

BAKED TROUT FILLET WITH ALMONDS

Preparation time: 10 minutes

Cooking times: 20 minutes

Doses for 4 people:

Ingredients:

Trout fillets: 4 (about 800g)

Flaked almonds: 50g

Lemon: 1, cut into thin slices

Fresh parsley: to taste

Salt and Pepper To Taste

Butter: 2 tablespoons

Preparation:

Preheat the oven to 180°C. Place the trout fillets on a baking tray lightly greased with butter. Season the fillets with salt, pepper and lemon slices. Distribute the flaked almonds evenly over the trout fillets. Add a few flakes of butter to the fillets. Bake for about 15/20 minutes or until the fish is cooked and the almonds are lightly golden. Serve the baked trout hot, garnished with chopped fresh parsley. Nutritional Values (per serving): Calories: 300 kcal Proteins: 25g Fat: 18g Carbohydrates: 5g Fibre: 2g Sugars: 1g Sodium: 400mg.

CHICKEN WITH HERBS WITH ASPARAGUS SIDE

Preparation time: 15 minutes

Cooking times: 25 minutes

Doses for 4 people:

Ingredients:

Chicken breast: 4 (about 600g)

Chopped fresh herbs

(rosemary, thyme, sage): 2 tablespoons

Lemon: 1, juice and grated zest

Garlic: 3 cloves, finely chopped

Asparagus: 500g, cleaned and cut

Extra virgin olive oil: 3 tablespoons

Salt and Pepper To Taste

Preparation:

Preheat the oven to 200°C. In a bowl, mix the chopped herbs, lemon juice and grated zest, minced garlic, salt, pepper and olive oil. Brush the chicken breast with the herb marinade on both sides. Place the chicken on a baking tray and cook in the oven for about 20/25 minutes or until completely cooked and golden. In the meantime, cook the asparagus by steaming or in boiling salted water for about 5/7 minutes, until they are tender but crunchy. Serve the herbed chicken hot, accompanied by asparagus. Nutritional Values (per serving): Calories: 350 kcal Proteins: 40g Fat: 15g Carbohydrates: 10g Fibre: 5g Sugars: 3g Sodium: 500mg

GRILLED CHICKEN WITH MEDITERRANEAN VEGETABLES

Preparation time: 20 minutes

Cooking times: 20 minutes

Doses for 4 people:

Ingredients:

Chicken breast: 4 (about 600g)

Courgettes: 2, cut into rounds

Eggplant: 2, diced

Peppers: 2, cut into strips

Tomatoes: 4, cut into wedges

Garlic: 3 cloves, finely chopped

Fresh basil: to taste

Extra virgin olive oil: 4 tablespoons

Salt and Pepper To Taste

Preparation:

Heat a grill or non-stick pan. Brush the chicken breasts lightly with olive oil and season with salt and pepper. Grill the chicken for about 5 to 7 minutes per side or until cooked through and golden brown. Meanwhile, in a pan, heat the olive oil and add the minced garlic. Add the chopped vegetables (zucchini, eggplant, peppers and tomatoes) and cook until tender but crunchy. Add fresh basil leaves and season with salt and pepper, if necessary. Serve the grilled chicken with Mediterranean vegetables. Nutritional Values (per serving): Calories: 380 kcal Proteins: 35g Fat: 18g Carbohydrates: 15g Fibre: 6g Sugars: 8g Sodium: 600mg.

TURKEY CURRY WITH VEGETABLES

Preparation time: 15 minutes

Cooking times: 25 minutes

Doses for 4 people:

Ingredients:

Sliced turkey breast: 600g

Mixed vegetables (courgettes, carrots, peppers):

500g, cut into cubes

Onion: 1, cut into thin slices

Garlic: 3 cloves, finely chopped

Curry powder: 2 tbsp

Coconut milk: 400ml

Extra virgin olive oil: 3 tablespoons

Salt and Pepper To Taste

Preparation:

In a large pan, heat the olive oil and sauté the onion and garlic until golden. Add the turkey slices and brown until well browned on both sides. Add the mixed vegetables and cook for a few minutes until tender but crunchy. Add the curry powder and mix well. Pour the coconut milk into the pan, bring to the boil, then reduce the heat and simmer for about 10 to 15 minutes until the sauce thickens. Season with salt and pepper to taste. Serve the turkey curry hot with brown rice or couscous. Nutritional Values (per serving): Calories: 380 kcal Proteins: 30g Fat: 20g Carbohydrates: 20g Fibre: 5g Sugars: 6g Sodium: 600mg

OMELETTE WITH SPINACH AND LOW HEATER CHEESE

Preparation time: 10 minutes

Cooking times: 15 minutes

Doses for 4 people:

Ingredients:

Eggs: 8

Fresh spinach: 200g, washed and cut

Diced low-fat cheese: 100g

Onion: 1, finely chopped

Extra virgin olive oil: 2 tablespoons

Salt and Pepper To Taste

Preparation:

In a non-stick pan, heat the olive oil and add the chopped onion. Fry until translucent. Add the washed and chopped fresh spinach and cook until wilted. In a bowl, beat the eggs with the diced low-fat cheese, salt and pepper. Pour the egg mixture over the spinach in the pan and cook over medium-low heat until the omelette is cooked through on the sides. Once the bottom part is well browned, turn the omelette with the help of a plate and cook the other side for a few minutes. Serve the omelette hot, cut into wedges. Nutritional Values (per serving): Calories: 220 kcal Proteins: 18g Fat: 12g Carbohydrates: 8g Fibre: 2g Sugars: 3g Sodium: 400mg.

STEAMED ASPARAGUS WITH LEMON AND ALMONDS SAUCE

Preparation time: 10 minutes

Cooking times: 10 minutes

Doses for 4 people:

Ingredients:

Asparagus: 500g, cleaned and cut

Flaked almonds: 50g

Lemon: 1, juice and

grated zest

Butter: 2 tablespoons (optional)

Salt and Pepper To Taste

Preparation:

In a steamer, bring water to a boil. Add the steamed asparagus and cook for about 5/7 minutes or until tender but crunchy. In the meantime, in a pan, lightly toast the flaked almonds. For the sauce, in a small bowl, combine the lemon juice, grated lemon zest, butter (if using), salt, and pepper. Arrange the asparagus on a serving plate and drizzle with the lemon sauce. Sprinkle the toasted almonds over the asparagus. Serve the steamed asparagus hot. Nutritional Values (per serving): Calories: 100 kcal Proteins: 4g Fat: 6g Carbohydrates: 8g Fibre: 4g Sugars: 2g Sodium: 200mg.

ROSEMARY CHICKEN WITH COURGETTE SIDE

Preparation time: 15 minutes

Cooking times: 25 minutes

Doses for 4 people:

Ingredients:

Chicken breast: 4 (about 600g)

Fresh rosemary sprigs: 4

Courgettes: 500g, cut into rounds

Garlic: 3 cloves, finely chopped

Extra virgin olive oil: 3 tablespoons

Salt and Pepper To Taste

Preparation:

Preheat the oven to 200°C. Season the chicken breasts with salt, pepper and rosemary leaves. In a pan, heat the olive oil and add the minced garlic. Fry until golden. Add the courgette slices and cook until tender but crunchy. Place the seasoned chicken breasts on a baking tray and cook in the oven for about 20/25 minutes or until they are well cooked and golden. Serve the rosemary chicken hot, accompanied by the courgettes. Nutritional Values (per serving): Calories: 280 kcal Proteins: 30g Fat: 12g Carbohydrates: 10g Fibre: 4g Sugars: 3g Sodium: 400mg.

CHICKEN CUTLET WITH ALMONDS AND LINSEEDS

Preparation time: 15 minutes

Cooking times: 15 minutes

Doses for 4 people:

Ingredients:

Chicken breast: 4 (about 600g)

Chopped almonds: 100g

Flaxseeds: 2 tablespoons

Eggs: 2, beaten

Flour: 50g

Extra virgin olive oil: 4 tablespoons

Salt and Pepper To Taste

Preparation:

Lightly press the chicken cutlets between two sheets of baking paper to make them thinner and more tender. In a bowl, mix the chopped almonds and flax seeds. Dip each chicken cutlet in the flour, then in the beaten eggs and finally in the almond and flaxseed mixture, pressing well to adhere. Heat the olive oil in a non-stick pan and cook the chicken cutlets for about 5/6 minutes per side or until they are golden brown and cooked. Drain them on absorbent paper to remove excess oil. Serve hot chicken cutlets with side dishes of your choice. Nutritional Values (per serving): Calories: 350 kcal Proteins: 35g Fat: 20g Carbohydrates: 10g Fibre: 5g Sugars: 2g Sodium: 400mg

GRILLED TUNA WITH LEMON SAUCE

Preparation time: 10 minutes

Cooking times: 10 minutes

Doses for 4 people:

Ingredients:

Fresh tuna fillets: 4 (about 800g)

Lemon: 2, juice and grated zest

Garlic: 2 cloves, finely chopped

Fresh parsley: 2

spoons, finely chopped

Extra virgin olive oil: 4 tablespoons

Salt and Pepper To Taste

Preparation:

In a bowl, mix the olive oil, lemon juice and grated zest, minced garlic, parsley, salt and pepper. Brush the tuna fillets with the prepared marinade. Heat a grill or non-stick pan and cook the tuna fillets for about 3/4 minutes per side or until cooked but still slightly pink inside. Serve the grilled tuna hot, accompanied by the lemon sauce. Nutritional Values (per serving): Calories: 280 kcal Proteins: 30g Fat: 15g Carbohydrates: 5g Fibre: 2g Sugars: 1g Sodium: 300mg.

BAKED SALMON WITH LEMON SAUCE AND HERB

Preparation time: 10 minutes

Cooking times: 20 minutes

Doses for 4 people:

Ingredients:

Salmon fillets: 4 (about 600g)

Lemon: 1, juice and grated zest

Garlic: 2 cloves, finely chopped

Fresh parsley: 2 tablespoons, finely chopped

Fresh thyme: 1 tablespoon, finely chopped

Extra virgin olive oil: 4 tablespoons

Salt and Pepper To Taste

Preparation:

Preheat the oven to 180°C. In a bowl, mix the olive oil, lemon juice and grated zest, minced garlic, parsley, thyme, salt and pepper. Place the salmon fillets on a baking tray lined with baking paper. Brush the salmon fillets with the prepared marinade. Bake in the oven for about 15/20 minutes or until the salmon is cooked and flakes easily with a fork. Serve the baked salmon hot, accompanied by the lemon and herb sauce. Nutritional Values (per serving): Calories: 300 kcal Proteins: 25g Fat: 18g Carbohydrates: 2g Fibre: 1g Sugars: 1g Sodium: 400mg

TURKEY MEATBALLS WITH CURRY

Preparation time: 15 minutes

Cooking times: 20 minutes

Doses for 4 people:

Ingredients:

Minced turkey meat: 500g

Onion: 1, finely chopped

Garlic: 2 cloves, finely chopped

Grated bread: 50g

Egg: 1, beaten

Curry powder: 2 tbsp

Extra virgin olive oil: 4 tablespoons

Salt and Pepper To Taste

Preparation:

In a bowl, mix the ground turkey with the onion, garlic, breadcrumbs, egg, curry powder, salt and pepper. Shape into meatballs with wet hands. Heat the olive oil in a non-stick pan and cook the turkey meatballs for about 10/12 minutes, turning them occasionally, until they are well cooked and golden. Drain them on absorbent paper to remove excess oil. Serve the curry turkey meatballs hot, accompanied by fresh side dishes. Nutritional Values (per serving): Calories: 250 kcal Proteins: 20g Fat: 12g Carbohydrates: 10g Fibre: 2g Sugars: 1g Sodium: 300mg.

VEAL CHOPS WITH GREEN PEPPER SAUCE

Preparation time: 15 minutes

Cooking times: 20 minutes

Doses for 4 people:

Ingredients:

Veal slices: 4 (about 600g)

Pickled green pepper: 2 tablespoons

Cooking cream: 200ml

Butter: 2 tablespoons

Salt and Pepper To Taste

Preparation:

Spread the veal slices with salt and pepper. In a pan, melt the butter and cook the veal slices until golden brown on both sides. Remove the slices from the pan and set aside. In the same pan, pour the cooking cream and green pepper. Cook over medium heat until the sauce thickens slightly. Put the veal slices back in the pan and heat them in the sauce for a few minutes. Serve the veal chops hot with the green pepper sauce. Nutritional Values (per serving): Calories: 350 kcal Proteins: 30g Fat: 20g Carbohydrates: 5g Fibre: 1g Sugars: 2g Sodium: 400mg

SOLE MUGNAIA STYLE WITH CAPERS AND LEMON

Preparation time: 10 minutes

Cooking times: 15 minutes

Doses for 4 people:

Ingredients:

Sole: 4 fillets (about 800g)

Flour: 50g

Butter: 4 tablespoons

Capers: 2 tablespoons, rinsed

Lemon: 1, juice and grated zest

Fresh parsley: 2

spoons, finely chopped

Salt and Pepper To Taste

Preparation:

Salt and pepper the sole fillets. Dredge the sole fillets in the flour, shaking off the excess. In a nonstick pan, melt the butter over medium-high heat. Add the sole fillets and cook for about 3/4 minutes per side, until golden and cooked. Add the capers, lemon juice and zest and parsley. Cook for another 2/3 minutes, gently turning the fillets to coat them with the sauce. Serve hot with lemon wedges and fresh parsley. Nutritional Values (per serving): Calories: 280 kcal Proteins: 25g Fat: 15g Carbohydrates: 10g Fibre: 2g Sugars: 1g Sodium: 400mg.

ROMAN-SRYLE ARTICHOKES

Preparation time: 20 minutes

Cooking times: 30 minutes

Doses for 4 people:

Ingredients:

Artichokes: 8 Large

Lemon: 1, juice

Fresh parsley: 4 tablespoons,

finely chopped

Garlic: 2 cloves, finely chopped

Extra virgin olive oil: 4 tablespoons

Salt and Pepper To Taste

Preparation:

Clean the artichokes, removing the tough outer leaves and cutting the tips. Cut the stems in half. Place the artichokes in a bowl of cold water with lemon juice to prevent oxidation. In a pan, heat the olive oil and add the chopped garlic and parsley. Add the artichokes to the pan and brown them lightly on both sides. Add water to cover the artichokes and let them cook over medium-low heat until they are soft. Serve hot, drizzled with a drizzle of olive oil and freshly ground black pepper. Nutritional Values (per serving): Calories: 120 kcal Proteins: 3g Fat: 7g Carbohydrates: 12g Fibre: 6g Sugars: 2g Sodium: 150mg

HERBS BEEF WITH ARUGULA AND TOMATOES SALAD

Preparation time: 15 minutes

Cooking times: 15 minutes

Doses for 4 people:

Ingredients:

Beef slices: 600g

Mix of fresh herbs (rosemary, thyme, parsley): 4 tablespoons, finely chopped

Garlic: 2 cloves, finely chopped

Arugula: 200g

Cherry tomatoes: 200g, cut in half

Extra virgin olive oil: 4 tablespoons

Balsamic vinegar: 2 tablespoons

Salt and Pepper To Taste

Preparation:

Season the beef slices with chopped fresh herbs, garlic, salt and pepper. Heat a non-stick pan and cook the beef slices for 2/3 minutes per side or until desired doneness. In a large bowl, mix the arugula and cherry tomatoes. Season the salad with olive oil, balsamic vinegar, salt and pepper. Serve the slices of beef hot with the Arugula and cherry tomato salad. Nutritional Values (per serving): Calories: 350 kcal Proteins: 30g Fat: 15g Carbohydrates: 10g Fibre: 3g Sugars: 5g Sodium: 250mg.

GRILLED PRAWNS WITH GARLIC AND PARSLEY SAUCE

Preparation time: 15 minutes

Cooking times: 5 minutes

Doses for 4 people:

Ingredients:

Fresh prawns: 500g,

shelled and cleaned

Garlic: 4 cloves, finely chopped

Fresh parsley: 4 tablespoons,

finely chopped

Lemon juice: 2 tablespoons

Extra virgin olive oil: 4 tablespoons

Salt and Pepper To Taste

Preparation:

In a large bowl, mix the minced garlic cloves, parsley, lemon juice, olive oil, salt and pepper. Add the shrimp to the marinade and mix well to coat them evenly. Leave the prawns to marinate in the refrigerator for at least 30 minutes. Preheat the grill and cook the marinated prawns for 2/3 minutes per side or until pink and well cooked. Serve the grilled prawns hot, accompanied by the garlic and parsley sauce. Nutritional Values (per serving): Calories: 180 kcal Proteins: 20g Fat: 8g Carbohydrates: 4g Fibre: 1g Sugars: 0g Sodium: 200mg

FISH FRITTERS WITH YOGURT SAUCE

Preparation time: 20 minutes

Cooking times: 10 minutes

Doses for 4 people:

Ingredients:

White fish fillets

(cod, hake, etc.):

500g, finely chopped

Eggs: 2

Breadcrumbs: 100g

Greek yogurt: 200g

Lemon juice: 2 tablespoons

Fresh herbs (parsley, chives):

4 tablespoons, finely chopped

Salt and Pepper To Taste

Preparation:

In a bowl, mix the chopped fish fillets, eggs, breadcrumbs, fresh herbs, salt and pepper. Form meatballs with the fish mixture. Heat some oil in a non-stick pan and fry the fishcakes until golden on both sides. In a bowl, mix the Greek yogurt with the lemon juice and a pinch of salt. Serve the fish fritters hot, accompanied by the yogurt sauce. Nutritional Values (per serving): Calories: 220 kcal Proteins: 25g Fat: 8g Carbohydrates: 12g Fibre: 1g Sugars: 2g Sodium: 250mg.

AUBERGINES STUFFED WITH QUINOA AND VEGETABLES

Preparation time: 20 minutes

Cooking times: 40 minutes

Doses for 4 people:

Ingredients:

Aubergine: Medium 4

Quinoa: 1 cup, cooked

Mixed vegetables (courgettes, peppers, carrots, etc.):

2 cups, diced

Onion: 1, chopped

Garlic: 2 cloves, finely chopped

Grated cheese: 1/2 cup

Fresh parsley: 2 tablespoons, finely chopped

Salt and Pepper To Taste

Extra virgin olive oil: 2 tablespoons

Preparation:

Cut the aubergines in half lengthwise and carefully empty them with a spoon. In a pan, heat the olive oil and fry the onion and garlic until golden. Add the mixed vegetables and cook until tender. Add the cooked quinoa, grated cheese, parsley, salt and pepper to the vegetable filling. Fill the aubergine halves with the prepared filling. Arrange the stuffed aubergines on a baking tray and cook in a preheated oven at 180°C for about 30 minutes or until the aubergines are tender. Serve hot. Nutritional Values (per serving): Calories: 220 kcal Proteins: 8g Fat: 6g Carbohydrates: 35g Fibre: 8g Sugars: 8g Sodium: 350mg

BEEF STEAK WITH BLACK PEPPER AND TOMATOES

Preparation time: 10 minutes

Cooking times: 10 minutes

Doses for 4 people:

Ingredients:

Beef steaks: 4

(about 200g each)

Ground black pepper: 2 tablespoons

Cherry tomatoes:

200g, cut in half

Extra virgin olive oil: 4 tablespoons

Salt to taste

Preparation:

Heat a non-stick pan over medium-high heat. Sprinkle both sides of the beef steaks with ground black pepper and a light sprinkle of salt. Add the steaks to the pan and cook for 3/4 minutes per side for rare, or longer depending on the desired doneness. During the last minutes of cooking, add the halved cherry tomatoes to the same pan to heat them slightly. Once cooked, transfer the steaks and cherry tomatoes to a serving platter. Season with a drizzle of extra virgin olive oil. Serve hot. Nutritional Values (per serving): Calories: 350 kcal Protein: 30g Fat: 18g Carbohydrates: 5g Fibre: 2g Sugars: 3g Sodium: 400mg.

VEGETABLE OMELETTE

Preparation time: 15 minutes

Cooking times: 15 minutes

Doses for 4 people:

Ingredients:

Eggs: 6

Mixed vegetables (courgettes, peppers, onions, tomatoes, etc.): 2 cups, diced

Grated cheese: 1/2 cup

Extra virgin olive oil: 2 tablespoons

Salt and Pepper To Taste

Preparation:

In a bowl, beat the eggs with the grated cheese, salt and pepper. In a non-stick pan, heat the olive oil and add the mixed vegetables. Cook until tender. Pour the beaten eggs over the vegetables and leave to cook over medium-low heat until the omelette is golden on the edges and compact. Using a lid or plate, turn the omelette and cook on the other side for another 5 minutes or until cooked through. Serve hot or at room temperature. Nutritional Values (per serving): Calories: 180 kcal Proteins: 12g Fat: 12g Carbohydrates: 6g Fibre: 2g Sugars: 3g Sodium: 300mg.

SHRIMP AND VEGETABLE SKEWERS

Preparation time: 20 minutes

Cooking times: 10 minutes

Doses for 4 people:

Ingredients:

Prawns: 16, peeled and cleaned

Mixed vegetables (peppers, onions, courgettes, tomatoes, etc.):

2 cups, cut into cubes

Extra virgin olive oil: 3 tablespoons

Lemon juice: 2 tablespoons

Salt and Pepper To Taste

Spices to taste (oregano, chili pepper, garlic powder, etc.)

Preparation:

Thread the prawns and vegetables onto skewers, alternating the ingredients. In a small bowl, mix the olive oil with the lemon juice, salt, pepper and spices to taste. Brush the skewers with the prepared marinade. Cook the skewers on a hot grill for 3/4 minutes per side or until the prawns are pink and the vegetables are tender. Serve hot, possibly accompanied by rice or salad. Nutritional Values (per serving): Calories: 220 kcal Proteins: 18g Fat: 10g Carbohydrates: 10g Fibre: 3g Sugars: 5g Sodium: 350mg.

TURKEY SCALLOPPINE WITH LEMON AND SAGE

Preparation time: 10 minutes

Cooking times: 15 minutes

Doses for 4 people:

Ingredients:

Turkey escalopes: 4

(about 150g each)

Lemon: 1, squeezed

Fresh sage leaves: 8

Vegetable broth: 1/2 cup

Extra virgin olive oil: 2 tablespoons

Salt and Pepper To Taste

Preparation:

In a nonstick skillet, heat the olive oil over medium-high heat. Add the turkey escalopes and brown them on both sides until golden. Add the lemon juice, sage leaves and vegetable broth. Reduce the heat and leave to cook for about 10 minutes or until the liquid has reduced and the scallops are tender. Season with salt and pepper according to taste. Serve hot, possibly accompanied by vegetables or side dishes of your choice. Nutritional Values (per serving): Calories: 250 kcal Proteins: 30g Fat: 10g Carbohydrates: 5g Fibre: 1g Sugars: 2g Sodium: 400mg

CHICKEN SAUSAGES WITH PEPPERS AND ONIONS

Preparation time: 15 minutes

Cooking times: 20 minutes

Doses for 4 people:

Ingredients:

Chicken sausages: 8

Mixed peppers (red, yellow, green): 2, cut into strips

Onions: 2, cut into slices

Extra virgin olive oil: 2 tablespoons

Salt and Pepper To Taste

Spices to taste (paprika, oregano, garlic powder, etc.)

Preparation:

In a nonstick skillet, heat the olive oil over medium heat. Add the chicken sausages and brown on both sides until well cooked. Add the onions and peppers to the same pan and cook until the vegetables are tender and lightly caramelized. Season with salt, pepper and spices to taste. Serve hot, possibly accompanied by mashed potatoes or salad. Nutritional Values (per serving): Calories: 320 kcal Proteins: 25g Fat: 18g Carbohydrates: 10g Fibre: 3g Sugars: 5g Sodium: 450mg.

BAKED TROUT FILLET WITH AROMATIC HERBS

Preparation time: 10 minutes

Cooking times: 20 minutes

Doses for 4 people:

Ingredients:

Trout fillets: 4 (about 150g each)

Fresh aromatic herbs

chopped (rosemary,

thyme, parsley): 2 tablespoons

Garlic: 2 cloves, minced

Lemon: 1, cut into thin slices

Extra virgin olive oil:

2 tbsp

Salt and Pepper To Taste

Preparation:

Preheat the oven to 180°C. Arrange the trout fillets on a baking tray lined with baking paper. Season the fillets with the chopped herbs, garlic, lemon juice, olive oil, salt and pepper. Cover the pan with aluminum foil and bake in the oven for about 15/20 minutes or until the fish is tender and flakes easily with a fork. Serve hot, possibly accompanied by side dishes of vegetables or potatoes. Nutritional Values (per serving): Calories: 180 kcal Proteins: 25g Fat: 8g Carbohydrates: 2g Fibre: 1g Sugars: 0g Sodium: 300mg.

GRILLED CHICKEN WITH TOMATO AND BASIL SALAD

Preparation time: 15 minutes

Cooking times: 15 minutes

Doses for 4 people:

Ingredients:

Chicken breast: 4

(about 150g each)

Tomatoes: 4, cut into slices

Fresh basil leaves: 1 bunch

Extra virgin olive oil: 3 tablespoons

Balsamic vinegar: 2 tablespoons

Salt and Pepper To Taste

Preparation:

Preheat the grill or griddle. Season the chicken breasts with salt, pepper and a drizzle of olive oil. Grill the chicken for about 6 to 7 minutes per side or until cooked through and has nice streaks from the grill. Meanwhile, prepare the tomato and basil salad: in a bowl, mix the tomato slices with the basil leaves, olive oil, balsamic vinegar, salt and pepper. Serve the hot chicken accompanied by the tomato and basil salad. Nutritional Values (per serving): Calories: 220 kcal Proteins: 30g Fat: 10g Carbohydrates: 5g Fibre: 2g Sugars: 3g Sodium: 350mg.

BAKED COD FILLET WITH OLIVES AND TOMATOES

Preparation time: 10 minutes

Cooking times: 20 minutes

Doses for 4 people:

Ingredients:

Cod fillets: 4

(about 150g each)

Cherry tomatoes:

200g, cut in half

Black olives: 1/2 cup, pitted

Garlic: 2 cloves, minced

Extra virgin olive oil: 3 tablespoons

Fresh parsley: 2 tablespoons, chopped

Salt and Pepper To Taste

Preparation:

Preheat the oven to 180°C. Arrange the cod fillets on a baking tray. Season the fish with salt, pepper, garlic, parsley, cherry tomatoes and olives. Drizzle with a drizzle of extra virgin olive oil. Bake in the oven for about 15/20 minutes or until the fish is tender and flakes easily with a fork. Serve hot, possibly accompanied by side dishes of vegetables or potatoes. Nutritional Values (per serving): Calories: 180 kcal Proteins: 25g Fat: 8g Carbohydrates: 5g Fibre: 2g Sugars: 3g Sodium: 300mg

CHICKEN WITH BLACK PEPPER SAUCE AND BROCCOLI SIDE DISH

Preparation time: 15 minutes

Cooking times: 25 minutes

Doses for 4 people:

Ingredients:

Chicken breast: 4

(approximately 160g each)

Broccoli: 1 bunch,

cleaned and cut into florets

Black peppercorns: 1 tbsp

Light heavy cream: 1/2 cup

Vegetable broth: 1/2 cup

Extra virgin olive oil: 2 tablespoons

Salt and Pepper To Taste

Preparation:

In a nonstick skillet, heat the olive oil over medium heat. Add the chicken breasts and cook on both sides until golden brown. Remove the chicken from the pan and set aside. In the same pan, add the black peppercorns and toast lightly. Add the vegetable broth and cooking cream, bring to the boil and reduce the liquid slightly. Add the chicken to the sauce and cook for an additional 5 minutes or until cooked through. Meanwhile, steam broccoli until tender but crisp. Serve the chicken with the black pepper sauce accompanied by the broccoli. Nutritional Values (per serving): Calories: 250 kcal Proteins: 30g Fat: 12g Carbohydrates: 7g Fibre: 3g Sugars: 2g Sodium: 350mg.

SIDE DISH RECIPES

SPINACH AND AVOCADO SALAD

Preparation time: 15 minutes

Cooking time: 0 minutes

Doses: 4 people

Ingredients:

200 g of fresh spinach

1 ripe avocado

100 g of cherry tomatoes

1/2 red onion, chopped

30 g of crumbled feta

20g pecans, chopped

Extra virgin olive oil

Balsamic vinegar

Salt and Pepper To Taste

Preparation:

Wash the spinach thoroughly and dry them with a cloth. Cut the avocado in half, remove the stone and peel, then cut the pulp into cubes. Cut the cherry tomatoes in half. In a large bowl, combine the spinach, avocado, cherry tomatoes, red onion, feta and pecans. Season with extra virgin olive oil, balsamic vinegar, salt and pepper to taste. Stir gently to combine all the ingredients. Serve the fresh and tasty salad immediately. Calories: Approximately 250 kcal, Fat: Approximately 15 g (of which 2 g saturated)

Carbohydrates: Approximately 10 g (of which 5 g fibre)

Protein: About 10 g

Vitamins: Vitamins A, C, K and folate

Minerals: Potassium, magnesium, iron and calcium

OVEN GRILLED VEGETABLES

Preparation time: 20 minutes

Cooking time: 30 minutes

Doses: 4 people

Ingredients:

2 peppers (red,

yellow or as desired)

1 courgette

1 aubergine

1 red onion

1 clove of garlic

Extra virgin olive oil

Aromatic herbs to taste

(basil, rosemary, thyme)

Salt and Pepper To Taste

Preparation:

Preheat the oven to 200°C. Wash and cut the vegetables into similar sized pieces. In a large bowl, combine the chopped vegetables, chopped garlic, extra virgin olive oil, aromatic herbs, salt and pepper to taste. Mix well to distribute the dressing over all the vegetables. Arrange the vegetables on a baking tray lined with baking paper. Bake in the oven for about 30 minutes, turning the vegetables halfway through cooking for even browning. Remove the grilled vegetables from the oven and serve them hot or warm as a side dish or complete vegetarian dish. Calories: Approximately 150 kcal, Fat: Approximately 10 g (of which 1 g is saturated)

Carbohydrates: Approximately 10 g (of which 5 g fibre)

Protein: About 5 g

Vitamins: Vitamins A, C, K and group B

BAKED CAULIFLOWER WITH TURMERIC

Preparation time: 20 minutes

Cooking time: 40 minutes

Doses: 4 people

Ingredients:

1 medium cauliflower

2 tablespoons extra virgin olive oil

1 teaspoon turmeric powder

1/2 teaspoon sweet paprika

1/4 teaspoon black pepper

Salt to taste

Sesame seeds to decorate (optional)

Preparation:

Preheat the oven to 200°C. Cut the cauliflower into florets and rinse them under running water. In a large bowl, combine the cauliflower florets, extra virgin olive oil, turmeric, paprika, black pepper and salt. Mix well to distribute the spices throughout the cauliflower. Arrange the cauliflower florets on a baking tray lined with baking paper. Bake in the oven for about 40 minutes, turning the florets halfway through cooking for even browning. Remove the baked cauliflower with turmeric and serve hot, decorating with sesame seeds to taste. Calories: Approximately 200 kcal, Fat: Approximately 12 g (of which 2 g saturated)

Carbohydrates: Approximately 20 g (of which 5 g fibre)

Protein: About 10 g

Vitamins: Vitamins A, C, K and group B

Minerals: Potassium, magnesium, manganese and calcium

STEAMED BROCCOLI WITH ALMONDS

Preparation time: 15 minutes

Cooking time: 10 minutes

Doses: 4 people

Ingredients:

1 medium broccoli

2 tablespoons extra virgin olive oil

1 clove garlic, minced

2 tablespoons lemon juice

30 g of flaked almonds

Salt and Pepper To Taste

Preparation:

Wash the broccoli and cut it into florets. Steam the broccoli for about 10 minutes, until tender but still crunchy. In a non-stick pan, heat the extra virgin olive oil and fry the chopped garlic for a minute. Add the flaked almonds and cook them for 2-3 minutes, stirring frequently, until they are golden and toasted. Add the steamed broccoli, lemon juice, salt and pepper to taste. Stir gently to combine all the ingredients. Serve steamed broccoli with almonds warm as a side dish or complete vegetarian dish. Calories: Approximately 180 kcal, Fat: Approximately 10 g (of which 2 g saturated)

Carbohydrates: Approximately 15 g (of which 5 g fibre)

Protein: About 10 g

Vitamins: Vitamins A, C, K and group B

Minerals: Potassium, magnesium, iron and calcium

LENTILS SALAD

Preparation time: 30 minutes

Cooking time: 20 minutes

Doses: 4 people

Ingredients:

200 g of dried lentils

1 red onion, chopped

1 green pepper, chopped

100g cherry tomatoes, cut in half

1 cucumber, cut into cubes

100g crumbled feta

Extra virgin olive oil

Balsamic vinegar

Lemon juice

Salt and Pepper To Taste

Preparation:

Rinse the lentils under running water. In a saucepan, cook the lentils in plenty of boiling water for about 20 minutes, or until tender. Drain the lentils and let them cool completely. In a large bowl, combine the cold lentils, chopped onion, chopped green pepper, cherry tomatoes, cucumber, crumbled feta and black olives (if using). Season with extra virgin olive oil, balsamic vinegar, lemon juice, salt and pepper to taste. Stir gently to combine all the ingredients. Serve the fresh and tasty lentil salad as a main dish or side dish. Calories: Approximately 350 kcal, Fat: Approximately 15 g (of which 3 g is saturated)

Carbohydrates: Approximately 40 g (of which 15 g fibre)

Protein: About 20 g

Vitamins: Vitamins A, C, K and group B

Minerals: Iron, magnesium, potassium and phosphorus

OVED STUFFED COURGETTES

Preparation time: 30 minutes

Cooking time: 40 minutes

Doses: 4 people

Ingredients:

4 medium courgettes

200g cooked brown rice, 150g ricotta

100g cherry tomatoes, cut in half

50 g of grated parmesan

1 red onion, chopped, 1 clove garlic, chopped, Fresh basil, chopped

Extra virgin olive oil, Salt and pepper to taste

Preparation:

Preheat the oven to 180°C. Wash the courgettes and cut them in half lengthwise, creating boats. With a spoon, remove the internal pulp of the courgettes, creating a

hollow. In a pan, non-stick, heat the extra virgin olive oil and fry the chopped onion for a minute. Add the minced garlic and cook for another minute, until fragrant. Add the courgette pulp removed previously, cut into cubes, and cook for 5 minutes, stirring frequently. Add the cooked brown rice, the tomato cut in half, the grated parmesan, the chopped basil, salt and pepper to taste. Mix well to combine all the ingredients. Fill the courgette boats with the rice and vegetable mixture. Arrange the stuffed courgettes on a baking tray lined with baking paper. Bake in the oven for about 40 minutes, or until the courgettes are tender and the filling is golden. Remove the stuffed courgettes from the oven and serve hot. Calories: Approximately 300 kcal, Fats: Approximately 15 g (of which 3 g are saturated), Carbohydrates: Approximately 30 g (of which 10 g fibre), Proteins: Approximately 15 g, Vitamins: Vitamins A, C, K and group B, Minerals: Potassium, magnesium, calcium and iron

CAULIFLOWER PUREE

Preparation time: 20 minutes

Cooking time: 20 minutes

Doses: 4 people

Ingredients:

1 medium cauliflower

1 medium potato

1 clove of garlic

200 ml of vegetable broth

2 tablespoons extra virgin olive oil

Salt and Pepper To Taste

Nutmeg to taste (optional)

Preparation:

Wash the cauliflower and cut it into florets. Peel the potato and cut it into chunks. In a pan, heat the extra virgin olive oil and fry the chopped garlic for a minute. Add the cauliflower florets and the diced potato, and cook for 5 minutes, stirring frequently. Pour in the vegetable broth and bring to the boil. Cover the pot and cook for about 20 minutes, or until the cauliflower and potato are very tender. Blend the mixture with a blender until you obtain a smooth and velvety cream. Season with salt, pepper and nutmeg to taste. Serve the cauliflower puree hot as a side dish or appetizer. Calories: Approximately 150 kcal, Fats: Approximately 5 g (of which 1 g saturated), Carbohydrates: Approximately 20 g (of which 5 g fibre), Proteins: Approximately 5 g, Vitamins: Vitamins A, C, K and group B

Minerals: Potassium, magnesium, manganese and calcium

QUINOA AND VEGETABLE SALAD

Preparation time: 20 minutes

Cooking time: 15 minutes

Doses: 4 people

Ingredients:

120 g of quinoa

200 g tomatoes, cut into cubes

1 cucumber, cut into cubes

1 green pepper, diced

100g crumbled feta

Black olives, pitted and

cut into rounds (optional)

Fresh basil, chopped

Extra virgin olive oil, Salt and pepper to taste

Balsamic vinegar, lemon juice

Preparation:

Rinse the quinoa under running water. In a saucepan, cook the quinoa in plenty of boiling water for about 15 minutes, or until tender. Drain the quinoa and let it cool completely. In a large bowl, combine the cold quinoa, diced tomatoes, diced cucumber, diced green pepper, crumbled feta and black olives (if using). Season with extra virgin olive oil, balsamic vinegar, lemon juice, salt and pepper to taste. Add the chopped basil and mix gently to combine all the ingredients. Serve the fresh and tasty quinoa and vegetable salad. Calories: Approximately 300 kcal, Fats: Approximately 12 g (of which 2 g saturated), Carbohydrates: Approximately 35 g (of which 5 g fibre), Proteins: Approximately 15 g, Vitamins: Vitamins A, C, K and group B

Minerals: Iron, magnesium, potassium and phosphorus

SAUTÉED BLACK CABBAGE WITH GARLIC AND LEMON

Preparation time: 15 minutes

Cooking time: 10 minutes

Doses: 4 people

Ingredients:

400 g of black cabbage

2 cloves garlic, minced

2 tablespoons extra virgin olive oil

Juice of 1 lemon

Salt and Pepper To Taste

Chopped fresh chili pepper (optional)

Preparation:

Wash the black cabbage and cut it into thin strips. In a non-stick pan, heat the extra virgin olive oil and fry the chopped garlic for a minute. Add the kale and cook for about 5 minutes, stirring frequently, until wilted. Add the lemon juice and cook for another minute. Season with salt, pepper and chilli to taste. Serve sautéed kale with garlic and hot lemon as a side dish or appetizer. Calories: Approximately 150 kcal

Fat: Approximately 8 g (of which 1 g is saturated)

Carbohydrates: Approximately 10 g (of which 5 g fibre)

Protein: About 5 g

Vitamins: Vitamins A, C, K and group B

Minerals: Potassium, magnesium, iron and calcium

ROASTED CARROTS WITH THYME

Preparation time: 15 minutes

Cooking time: 40 minutes

Doses: 4 people

Ingredients:

500 g of carrots

2 tablespoons extra virgin olive oil

1 clove garlic, minced

1 sprig of fresh thyme

Salt and Pepper To Taste

Preparation:

Preheat the oven to 200°C. Peel the carrots and cut them into rounds about 1 cm thick. In a large bowl, combine the carrots, extra virgin olive oil, chopped garlic, fresh thyme, salt and pepper to taste. Mix well to distribute the seasoning

on all the carrots. Arrange the carrots on a baking tray lined with baking paper. Bake in the oven for about 40 minutes, turning the carrots halfway through cooking for even browning. Remove the roasted carrots with thyme from the oven and serve hot. Tips: You can add other flavors to roasted carrots, such as rosemary, paprika or cumin. For a more intense flavor, you can marinate the carrots in the dressing for at least 30 minutes before cooking them in the oven. (per portion of approximately 200g): Calories: Approximately 180 kcal, Fat: Approximately 10 g (of which 1 g is saturated) Carbohydrates: Approximately 25 g (of which 5 g fibre), Protein: Approximately 2 g

Vitamins: Vitamin A: 280% of the (VGR) Vitamin C: 30% of the VGR Vitamin K: 150% of the VGR

Minerals: Potassium: 500 mg (14% of VGR) Manganese: 1.5 mg (8% of VGR) Fibre: 5 g (20% of VGR)

CONCLUSION

In conclusion, the Low Glycemic Index Diet 2025 presents itself as an extraordinary path to optimal health and overall well-being. By thoroughly understanding the glycemic index and its impact on metabolic health, we have opened the door to a new perspective on nutrition. This book has provided not only a detailed overview of the glycemic index but also a practical guide to successfully implementing this approach into your daily life. From delicious, nutritious recipes to balanced meal plans, you now have the tools you need to make informed food decisions.

Weight management becomes an exciting challenge, where every meal is an opportunity to nourish the body intelligently. The variety of culinary options presented makes a flexible approach possible, suitable for different preferences and lifestyles. We have addressed the common challenges that may arise during this journey and provided Always remember that this is not just a temporary change, but a lasting investment in your health. Staying motivated is key, and the book has provided you with ongoing inspiration to tackle every step of the way with confidence. Ultimately, the Glycemic Index Diet is not just a dietary guide, but a travel companion for a healthier and more fulfilling life. Take control of your food choices, nourish your body with intention, and enjoy the benefits of a balanced, energized life.

Thank you for embarking on this journey with us, and may you enjoy the fruits of your new adventure towards lasting health and well-being. The recipes, designed with care and creativity, make every meal a unique culinary experience. In conclusion, the 2025 Glycemic Index Diet is more than just a book; it is a manifesto for positive change. The author, with competence and passion, demonstrates that every food choice can be a step towards a healthier life for ourselves and for the world we call home. An essential read for anyone who wants to nourish their body and contribute to a sustainable future.

Thank you, for this nourishing inspiration that goes beyond the plate. If the book has inspired you, helped you in any way, I would be infinitely grateful if you could take a moment to leave a review. Your words could be a guiding light for other wellness seekers embarking on this path. I thank you deeply for choosing The Low Glycemic Index Diet 2025" as your travel companion towards a healthier and more conscious life. With gratitude,

[KLARLOCK]